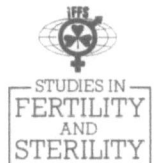

STUDIES IN
FERTILITY
AND
STERILITY

Research
in
Family
Planning

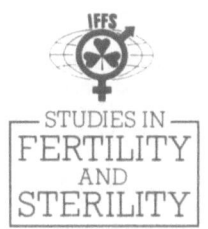

STUDIES IN
FERTILITY
AND
STERILITY

Research
in
Family
Planning

Edited by
J. Bonnar, W. Thompson
and R. F. Harrison

Themes from the XIth World Congress on Fertility and Sterility,
Dublin, June 1983, held under the Auspices of the International
Federation of Fertility Societies

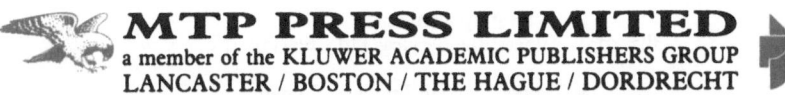

MTP PRESS LIMITED
a member of the KLUWER ACADEMIC PUBLISHERS GROUP
LANCASTER / BOSTON / THE HAGUE / DORDRECHT

Published in the UK and Europe by
MTP Press Limited
Falcon House
Lancaster, England

British Library Cataloguing in Publication Data

Research in family planning.—(Studies
in fertility and sterility)
1. Contraception
I. Bonnar, J.   II. Thompson, W.
III. Harrison, R. F.   IV. Series
613.9′4   RG136

ISBN-13:978-94-010-8971-5   e-ISBN-13:978-94-009-5604-9
DOI: 10.1007/978-94-009-5604-9

Published in the USA by
MTP Press
A division of Kluwer Boston Inc
190 Old Derby Street
Hingham, MA 02043, USA

Library of Congress Cataloging in Publication Data

Main entry under title:
World Congress of Fertility and Sterility (11th: 1983:
Dublin, Dublin)
Research in family planning.

(Studies in fertility and sterility)
Includes bibliographies and index.
1. Contraception – Congresses. 2. Birth control –
Congresses. 3. Fertility, Human – Congresses. 4.
Infertility, Female – Congresses. I. Bonnar, John. II.
Thompson, W. III. Harrison, R. F. (Robert
Frederick) IV. International Federation of Fertility
Societies. V. Series.
RG136.W69   1983   613.9′4   85-17170

Phototypesetting by
Blackpool Typesetting Services Ltd., Blackpool

Butler & Tanner Limited, Frome and London

Contents

v

CONTENTS

Preface

This volume contains the papers on family planning research which were presented at the XIth World Congress on Fertility and Sterility held in Dublin, Ireland in June, 1983 under the auspices of the International Federation of Fertility Societies. These papers were presented during the related communications sessions of the Congress and have been brought together into a special volume which will be of major interest to those concerned with family planning.

Section 1, deals with the area of natural family planning, determination of the fertile period and effects of lactation. Steroid contraception, vaginal and intrauterine contraception, abortion and sterilization are included in Sections 2–4. Social aspects of fertility control are covered in Section 5 and the final section contains studies of the effects of gossypol as a male contraceptive. This volume brings together important new knowledge in the area of family planning, clarifies some of the problems and should stimulate research on the many unresolved issues in this vitally important area.

John Bonnar
Robert F. Harrison
William Thompson
Dublin 1984

List of Contributors

H. ABUDEJAJA
Family & Community Medicine
Faculty of Medicine
University of Garyounis
PO Box 1451, Benghazi
LIBYA

A. O. ADEKUNLE
Department of Obstetrics & Gynaecology
University College Hospital
Ibaden
NIGERIA

T. S. BAKER
Research & Development
Boots-Celltech Diagnostics Ltd
240 Bath Road
Slough SL1 4ET
UNITED KINGDOM

B. N. BARWIN
Gynecoloy + Infertility
770 Broadview Avenue, Suite B-1
Ottawa, Ont K2A 3Z3
CANADA

S. BORTOLUSSI
1st Chair Gynaecology
University of Buenos Aires
Arendles 3,300 (1425)
Buenos Aires
ARGENTINA

P. X. J. M. BOUCKAERT
Department of Obstetrics & Gynaecology
De Wever Hospital
PO Box 4446
6401 CX Heerlen
THE NETHERLANDS

B. N. CHAKRAVARTY
Department of Obstetrics & Gynaecology
NRS Medical College
Calcutta
INDIA

S. CHATTOPADLYAY
BR Singh Hospital
Calcutta
INDIA

W. P. COLLINS
Department of Obstetrics & Gynaecology
Kings College Hospital
Denmark Hill
London SE5 8RX
UNITED KINGDOM

W. F. COULSON
Courtauld Institute of Biochemistry
The Middlesex Hospital Medical School
Cleveland Street
London W1P 7PN
UNITED KINGDOM

M. COUTINCHO
Maternidade Climerio de Oliveira
Rua do Limoeiro
No 1-Nazare
Salvador 40.000 Bahia
BRAZIL

A. CUCCI
Department Laboratory Analysis
Hospital Maggiore C. A. Pizzardi
via Nigrisoli
40100 Bologna
ITALY

S. DEGANI
Department of Obstetrics & Gynecology
Haifa Medical Center (Rothschild)
Faculty of Medicine, Technion
47 Golomb Street
PO Box 4940
Haifa 31048
ISRAEL

Z. DELATOLA
Areteion University Hospital
Department of Bacteriology
76 Vass Sofias Avenue
Athens 611
GREECE

K. DE VRIES
Department of Obstetrics & Gynecology
Haifa Medical Center (Rothschild)
Faculty of Medicine, Technion
47 Golomb Street
PO Box 4940
Haifa 31048
ISRAEL

R. DI MICCO
Department of Obstetrics & Gynecology
Hospital "Maggiore" C. A. Pizzardi
Div Obstetrics & Gynecology "Maternita"
Via D'Azelgio 56
Bologna 40123
ITALY

I. EIBSCHITZ
Department of Obstetrics & Gynecology
Haifa Medical Center (Rothschild)
Faculty of Medicine, Technion
47 Golomb Street
PO Box 4940
Haifa 31048
ISRAEL

R. ERNY
Gynecologie-Obstetrique
Hôpital La Conception
144 Rue Saint Pierre
13005 Marseille
FRANCE

J. J. ETCHEPAREBORDA
Department of Gynaecology
University of Buenos Aires
Arenales 3,300 (1425)
Buenos Aires
ARGENTINA

EL. S. ETMAN
Department of Obstetrics & Gynecology
Misr Co's Hospital
Mehalla El Kubra
EGYPT

A. M. FLYNN
Department of Obstetrics & Gynaecology
University of Birmingham
Birmingham Maternity Hospital
Edgbaston
Birmingham B15 2TG
UNITED KINGDOM

H. FRANGEHHEIM
Department of Gynecology & Obstetrics
Städtische Frauenklinik
D775 Konstanz
WEST GERMANY

V. FRYGANA
Areteion University Hospital
Department of Bacteriology
76 Vass Sofias Avenue
Athens 611
GREECE

G. GAHN
Zentrum für Gynäkologie und Geburtshilfe
der J. W. Goethe-Universität
Abteilung für gynäkologische Endokrinologie
Theodor Stern-Kai 7
D-6000 Frankfurt/Main
WEST GERMANY

R. GAMBRELL
Department of Endocrinology
Medical College of Georgia
Augusta
Georgia 30912
USA

U. J. GASPARD
Department of Obstetrics & Gynaecology
State University of Liège
81, Bd de la Constitution
B4020 Liège
BELGIUM

R. GIMES
I. Department of Obstetrics & Gynaecology
Semmelweiss University
Budapest
Budapest 1088 Baross u 27
HUNGARY

LIST OF CONTRIBUTORS

N. GOLDSTUCK
Marie Stopes House
Well Woman Centre
London W1P GBE
UNITED KINGDOM

W. GROSS
Gustav Embden-Zentrum der Biologischen
Chemi der J. W. Goethe-Universität
Theodor Stern-Kai 7
D-6000 Frankfurt/Main
WEST GERMANY

W. GRÜNBERGER
Ist Department Obstetrics & Gynaecology
University of Vienna
Spitalgasse 23
A1090 Vienna
AUSTRIA

A. A. HASPELS
Department of Obstetrics & Gynaecology
State University Hospital
Catharinesingel 101
3511 GV Utrecht
THE NETHERLANDS

L. HEISTERBERG
Department of Gynecology
Bispebjerg Hospital
DK-2400 Copenhagen NV
DENMARK

R. J. HOLDSWORTH
Research & Development
Boots-Celltech Diagnostics Ltd
240 Bath Road
Slough S21 4ET
UNITED KINGDOM

T. HOMONNAI
Andrology Institute for the Study of Fertility
Serlin Maternity Hospital, Hakirya, Tel-Aviv
Tel-Aviv PO Box 7079
ISRAEL 61070

H. HONJO
Department of Obstetrics & Gynecology
Kyoto Prefectural University of Medicine
Kawaramachi Hirokoji
Kamikyo-ku
Kyoto 602
JAPAN

H. HOSHIAI
Department of Obstetrics & Gynecology
Tohoku University School of Medicine
1-1 Seiryomachi
Sendai 980
JAPAN

T. KASEKI
Kaseki Hospital
Sakae 4-16-16
Naka-ku
Nagoya 460
JAPAN

E. KESSERÜ
1st Chair Gynaecology
University of Buenos Aires
Arenales 3,300 (1425)
Buenos Aires
ARGENTINA

J. KITAWAKI
Department of Obstetrics & Gynecology
Kyoto Prefectural University of Medicine
Kawaramachi Hirokoji
Kamikyo-ku
Kyoto 602
JAPAN

U. J. KOCH
Freie Universität Berlin
Bismarckstrasse 67
D-1000 Berlin 39
WEST GERMANY

E. KOUMENDAKOU
Areteion University Hospital
Department of Bacteriology
76 Vass Sofias Avenue
Athens 611
GREECE

H. KUHL
Zentrum für Gynäkologie und Geburtshilfe
  der J. W. Goethe-Universität
Abteilung für gynäkologische Endokrinologie
Theodor Stern Kai 7
D-6000 Frankfurt/Main
WEST GERMANY

K. H. KURZ
IRIR
International Institute for Reproduction
Kaiser-Wilhelm-Ring 22
D-4000 Dusseldorf
WEST GERMANY

G. LADA
II Department of Medicine
Semmelweis University
Budapest 1088 Szentkiralyi u 46
HUNGARY

M. M. LEGNAIN
Department of Obstetrics & Gynaecology
Faculty of Medicine
University of Garyounis
Benghazi
LIBYA

F. LEIDENBERGER
I.R.I.R.
International Institute for Reproduction
Kaiser-Wilhelm-ring 22
D-4000 Dusseldorf
WEST GERMANY

L. LEVITAN
Department of Obstetrics & Gynecology
Haifa Medical Center (Rothschild)
Faculty of Medicine, Technion
47 Golomb Street
PO Box 4940 Haifa 31048
ISRAEL

M. LEVRIER
Gynecologie-Endocrinologie
24 Ave du Mal de Lattre de Tarrisgny
33600 Talence
FRANCE

A. S. LUYCKX
Department of Clinical Pharmacology
Institute of Medicine
State University of Liège
66 Bd de la Constitution
B 4020 Liège
BELGIUM

R. C. MAIER
Department of Obstetrics & Gynecology
Wilford Hall USAF Medical Center
Lackland AFB Texas 78236
USA

W. MÄRZ
Gustav Embden-Zentrum der Biologischen
Chemi der J. W. Goethe-Universität
Theodor Stern-Kai 7
D-6000 Frankfurt/Main
WEST GERMANY

H. G. MASSOURAS
Areteion University Hospital
Obstetrics & Gynaecology Department
3 Marasli Street
Athens 106 76
GREECE

P. MEIER-OEHLKE
I.R.I.R.
International Institute for Reproduction
Kaiser-Wilhelm-Ring 22
D-4000 Düsseldorf
WEST GERMANY

R. MORI
Department of Obstetrics & Gynecology
Tohoku University School of Medicine
1-1 Seiryocho, Sendai 980
JAPAN

F. NAGAIKE
Department of Obstetrics & Gynecology
Tohoku University School of Medicine
1-1 Seiryocho, Sendai 980
JAPAN

T. NAMBARA
Pharmaceutical Institute
Tohoku University
Aza-Aoba Aramaki, Sendai 980
JAPAN

M. J. O'DOWD
Department of Obstetrics & Gynaecology
Portiuncula Hospital
Ballinasloe, Co Galway
IRELAND

H. OKADA
Department of Obstetrics & Gynecology
Kyoto Prefectural University of Medicine
Kawaramachi Hirokoji, Kamikyo-ku
Kyoto 602
JAPAN

N. PARIKH
Gynaecology Obstetrics & Family Planning
Nowrosjee Wadia Maternity Hospital
Acharya Donde Marg, Parel
Bombay 400 012
INDIA

A. PARUCH
Department of Obstetrics & Gynaecology
Al-Jamahiriya Hospital
Benghazi
LIBYA

LIST OF CONTRIBUTORS

R. PATTON
Department of Obstetrics & Gynaecology
Portiuncula Hospital
Ballinasloe, Co Galway
IRELAND

F. PAZ
Biology of Reproduction
Institute for the Study of Fertility
Serlin Maternity Hospital
Hakirya, Tel Aviv
PO Box 7079
ISRAEL 61070

K. PETERSEN
Department of Obstetrics & Gynecology YB
Rigshospitalet
DK-2100 Copenhagen Ø
DENMARK

A. E. PONTIROLI
Direzione Medica "Farmitalia-Carloerba"
Via C. Imbonati
Milano
ITALY

W. PRENDIVILLE
Academic Department of Obstetrics
& Gynaecology
Bristol Maternity Hospital
St Michael's Hill
Bristol B52 8EG
UNITED KINGDOM

H. H. RIEDEL
Department of Obstetrics and Gynecology
University of Kiel
23 Kiel Hegewischstrasse 4
WEST GERMANY

G. ROMBERG
Zentrum für Gynäkologie und Geburtshilfe
der J. W. Goethe-Universität
Abteilung für Gynakologische
Endokrinologie
Theodor Stern-Kai 7
D-6000 Frankfurt/Main
WEST GERMANY

M. A. ROMUS
Department of Obstetrics & Gynaecology
State University of Liège
81 Bd de la Constitution
B 4020 Liège
BELGIUM

P. ROYSTON
Department of Computing & Statistics
MRC Clinical Research Centre
Harrow
Middlesex
UNITED KINGDOM

H. N. SALLAM
Department of Obstetrics & Gynaecology
Womens Hospital, St Lukes Medical Center
Amsterdam Avenue, 114th Street, New York
N.Y. 10025
USA

A. SARTANI
Direzione Medica "Famitalia-Carloerba"
Vai C Imbonati
Milano
ITALY

J. H. SCHADE
Nuclear Medicine
Clinical Chemistry Laboratory
Jelsumerstraat 6
8917 EN Leeuwarden
HOLLAND

L. A. SCHELLEKENS
Department of Obstetrics & Gynaecology
De Wever Hospital
PO Box 4446
6401 CX Heerlen
THE NETHERLANDS

L. E. M. SCHIPORST
Department of Obstetrics & Gynaecology
Kings College Hospital
Denmark Hill
London SE5 8RX
UNITED KINGDOM

K. SEMM
Department of Obstetrics and Gynecology
University of Kiel
Hegewischestrasse 4
D-2300 Kiel
WEST GERMANY

M. SHARI
Department of Obstetrics and Gynecology
Haifa Medical Center (Rothschild)
Faculty of Medicine, Technion
47 Golomb Street
PO Box 4940
Haifa 31048
ISRAEL

V. SILVA
Maternidade Climerio de Oliveira
Rua do Limoeiro No 1-Nazare
Salvador Bahia 40.000
BRAZIL

R. SINGH
Department of Family & Community
  Medicine
Faculty of Medicine
University of Garyounis
Benghazi
LIBYA

R. SNOWDEN
Institute of Population Studies
University of Exeter
Hoopern House
101 Pennsylvania Road
Exeter EX4 63T
Devon
UNITED KINGDOM

G. SPINOLA
Centre de Recherches en Endocrinologie
Moléculaire
Le Centre Hospitalier de l'Université Laval
2705 Blvd Laurier
Québec G1V 4G2
CANADA

J. SPONA
Department of Molecular Endocrinology
First Department of Obstetrics &
  Gynecology
University of Vienna
Spitalgasse 23
A-1090 Vienna
AUSTRIA

M. SUZUKI
Department of Obstetrics & Gynecology
Tohoku University School of Medicine
1-1 Seiryocho
Sendai 980
JAPAN

H. D. TAUBERT
Zentrum fur Gynakologie und Geburtshilfe
  der J. W. Goethe-Universitat
Abteilung fur gynakologische Endokrinologie
Theodor Stern Kai 7
D-6000 Frankfurt/Main
WEST GERMANY

R. THAU
The Population Council
Center for Biomedical Research
1230 York Avenue
New York
N.Y. 10021
USA

M. THIERY
Department of Obstetrics & Gynecology
Academic Hospital
University of Gent
De Pintelaan 185
9000 Gent
BELGIUM

A. TSUIKI
Department of Obstetrics & Gynaecology
Tohoku University School of Medicine
1-1 Seiryocho
Sendai 980
JAPAN

S. UEHARA
Department of Obstetrics & Gynecology
Tohoku University School of Medicine
1-1 Seoryocho
Sendai 980
JAPAN

M. F. H. A. VAN DER CRUYS
Department of Microbiology
De Wever Hospital
PO Box 4446
6401 CX Heerlen
THE NETHERLANDS

H. VAN DER PAS
Obstetrics & Gynecology
St Elisabeth Ziekenhuis
2300 Turnhout
BELGIUM

W. VAN OS
Department of Obstetrics & Gynecology
Elisabeth Gasthuis
PO 417
2000 AK Haarlem
THE NETHERLANDS

M. R. VAN SANTEN
Department of Obstetrics & Gynaecology
Dijkzigt University Hospital
Dr Molewaterplein 40
3015 GD Rotterdam
THE NETHERLANDS

LIST OF CONTRIBUTORS

L. VIDELA-RIVERO
1st Chair Gynaecology
University of Buenos Aires
Arenales 3,300 (1425)
Buenos Aires
ARGENTINA

Y. YAOI
Department of Obstetrics & Gynaecology
Koshigaya Hospital
School of Medicine
Dokkyo University, 50-1-2 Chome
Minami-Koshigaya-shi
Saitama-Ken (343)
JAPAN

J. YASUDA
Department of Obstetrics & Gynecology
Kyoto Prefectural University of Medicine
Kawaramachi Hirokoji, Kamikyo-ku
Kyoto 602
JAPAN

E. ZANARDI
Department of Obstetrics & Gynaecology
Hospital "Maggiore" C. A. Pizzardi
II Div Obstetrics & Gynaecology
   "Maternita"
via D'Azelglio 56
40123 Bologna
ITALY

A. ZIMMERMAN
Japan Family Life Association
Yuwa Building
Shiba 3-4-16
Minato-ku
Tokyo 105
JAPAN

Section 1

Natural Family Planning, the Fertile Period and Lactation

1

The reliability of women's subjective assessment of the fertile period relative to urinary gonadotrophins and follicular ultrasonic measurements during the menstrual cycle

A. M. FLYNN, M. DOCKER, R. MORRIS, S. LYNCH AND J. P. ROYSTON

INTRODUCTION

There has been an increased interest in Natural Family Planning (NFP) in recent years. In practice, NFP requires that the fertile days in the cycle can be identified by the woman herself, so that pregnancies can be achieved or avoided by planned sexual intercourse. Consequently, to ensure success with these methods it is important to assess the reliability of the clinical indices used to detect the fertile time.

The introduction of high-resolution ultrasound scanners offers a precise method of timing ovulation and the fertile period[1]. This study was designed to compare the clinical and hormonal indicators of fertility with a presumed fertile period derived from the ultrasonic detection of ovulation.

SUBJECTS AND METHODS

Subjects

The study was carried out in eight healthy fertile women whose ages ranged from 25 to 35 years, and who were experienced users of the sympto-thermal method of NFP. Table 1 shows the data collected from these women.

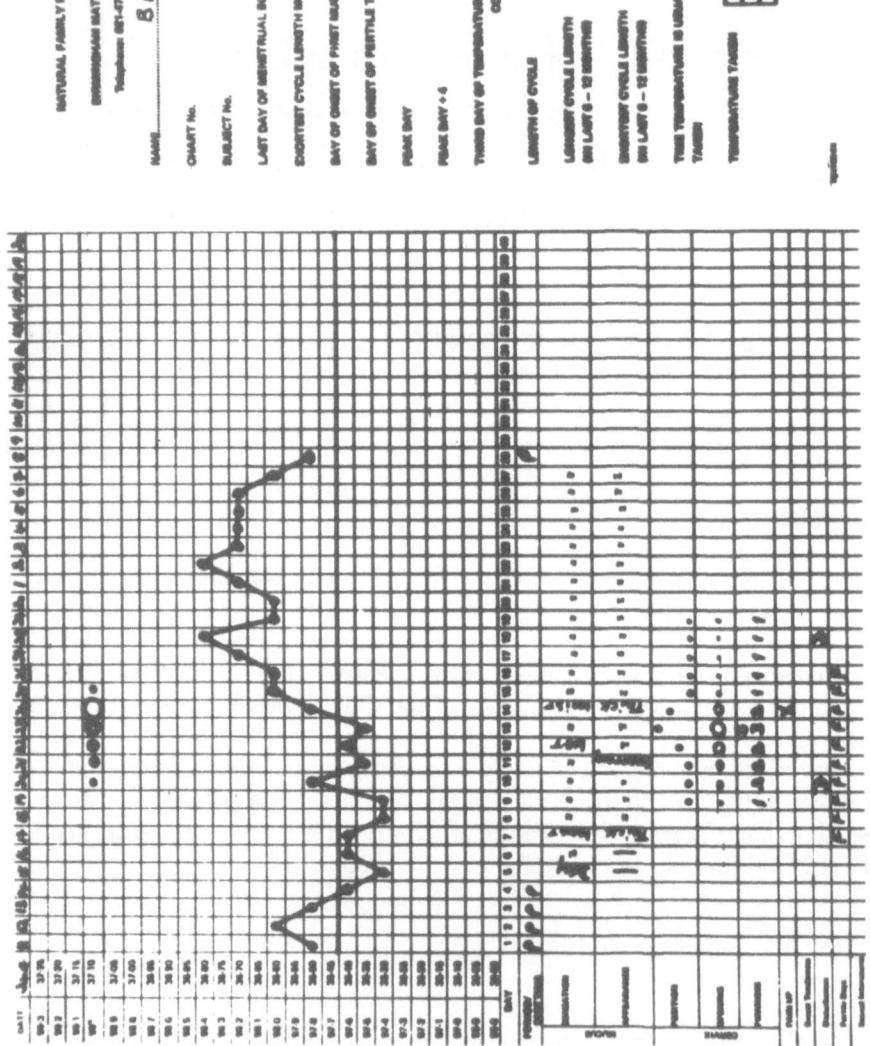

Figure 1 Sympto-thermal chart

4

Table 1 Data collected from the women

Subjects	Cycles contributed	Sympto-thermal charts	Hormonal data	Ultrasonic measurements
8	25	25	23	23

Sympto-thermal chart
The women made a subjective assessment of their fertile time by observing and charting changes in basal body temperature, cervical mucus and the uterine cervix, ovulation pain and breast symptoms. From these indices they deduced their probable fertile days for the cycle. Figure 1 shows one of these completed charts.

Hormone assays
All hormone assays were measured in specimens of early morning urine (EMU) collected daily by the women, and stored in their deep freezers until transferred to the laboratory for assay. Oestrone-3-glucuronide (E_1-3-G) and pregnanediol-3α-glucuronide (Pd-3d-G) were measured by the method described by Collins[2], FSH and LH were estimated by double antibody radioimmunoassays using reagents described by Lynch and Shirley[3].

Ultrasonic measurements
These were performed with the ATL Mk III ultrasound scanner which has a 3 mega Hertz (MHz) mechanical sector probe. Scanning was begun on the day of the cycle which the women estimated to be the beginning of their fertile period, it was continued on a daily basis with intervals of 24 hours, until maximum follicular growth of the dominant follicle was attained with subsequent follicular rupture and disappearance.

Definitions

The day of maximum follicular growth + 1 was considered to be the *day of ovulation* (marked 0 on the figures).

A *probable fertile time* was estimated to be − 5 to + 1 from day 0.

The following five indices were used to estimate the *beginning of the fertile period*:

(1) The shortest length of the last six menstrual cycles − 19 (S − 19).
(2) The first day of appearance of any mucus.
(3) The first day of appearance of fertile-type mucus.
(4) The day of the first significant rise in E_1-3-G.
(5) The day of the first significant rise in the ratio E_1-3-G/Pd-3α-G.

The indicators used to detect *the end of the fertile period were:*
  (1) The first day of the BBT rise + 2.
  (2) The peak mucus day + 3.
  (3) The day of peak E_1-3-G + 3.

RESULTS

Ovulation was presumed to have occurred by ultrasonic measurements in the 23 cycles in which these measurements were made. Sympto-thermal charts indicated ovulation in all 25 cycles. Hormonal data was available for 23 cycles. In two cycles the specimens were poorly labelled and these cycles are not included in the results.

There was one conceptional cycle for which clinical, hormonal and ultrasonic data were complete.

The mean length and range of the follicular and luteal phases are shown in Table 2.

Table 2 Mean length and range of the follicular and luteal phases of the menstrual cycle

	Mean (days)	Range (days)
Follicular phase	14.2	8–22
Luteal phase	13.2	10–17

Figure 2 is a histogram showing the temporal relationship of these clinical indicators used to detect the beginning of the fertile period to a fertile time derived from ultrasonic detection of ovulation.

If one used the calendar calculation S-19 only two of the 23 cycles fell within the ultrasonic fertile period. Using the first day of the appearance of any mucus six of the 23 cycles fell within the ultrasonic fertile period. When one used the first day of the appearance of fertile-type mucus, 20 of the 23 cycles fell within the ultrasonic fertile period.

Figure 3 is a histogram showing the temporal relationship for the first significant rise of the hormone E_1-3-G, and the ratio E_1-3-G/Pd-3α-G to the derived fertile period. Using the day of the first significant rise in E_1-3-G, 15 of the 23 cycles fell within the ultrasonic fertile period, whereas when one used the day of the first significant rise in the ratio only nine of the 23 cycles fell within the ultrasonic fertile period.

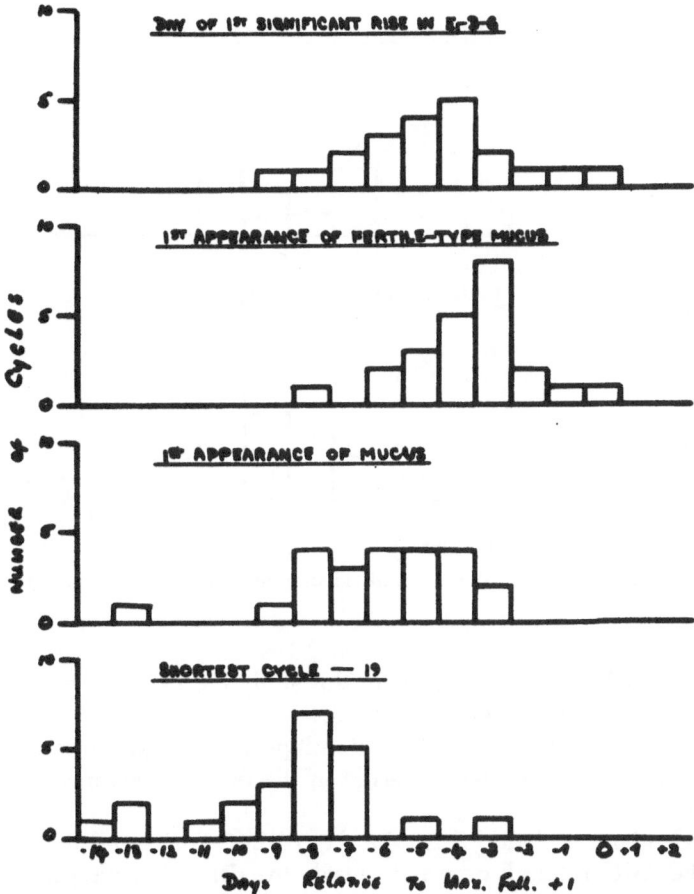

Figure 2 Temporal relationship of three clinical indicators to the beginning of the derived fertile time

Figure 4 is a histogram showing the temporal relationship between the clinical and chemical indicators of the end of the fertile time and the fertile period derived from ultrasonic measurements.

When one used the first day of BBT rise + 2, 20 of the 23 cycles occurred outside the derived fertile period.

There is some uncertainty about the temporal relationship in the three cycles where the BBT rise occurred on day − 1. They could be considered borderline although by our definition they fell within the fertile time.

Using the day of peak mucus + 3, 22 of the 23 cycles fell outside the derived fertile period. Using the chemical indicator peak E_1-3-G, 21 of the 23 cycles fell outside the derived fertile period. Out of 21 cycles where an LH peak was

7

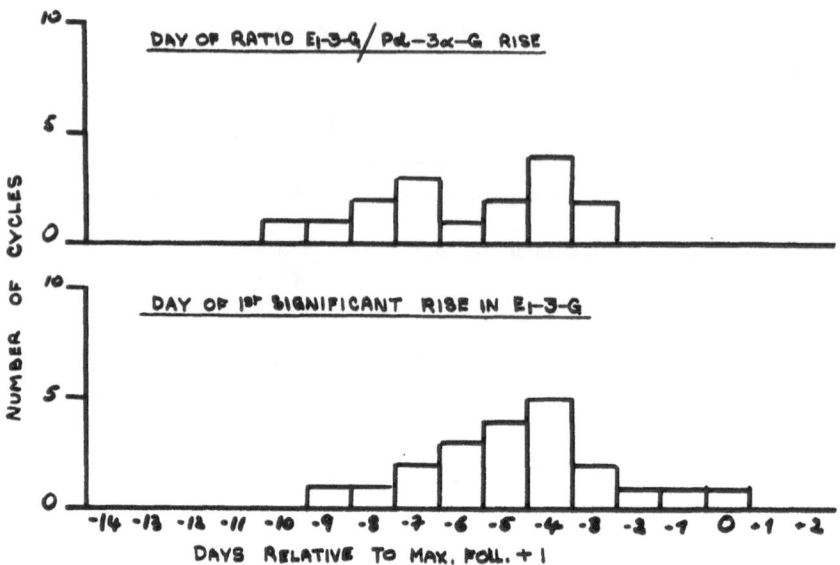

Figure 3　Temporal relationship of two chemical indicators to the beginning of the derived fertile time

detected, 17 fell on day 0 or later. In this study the LH peak proved a poor detector of the ovulatory event.

Figure 5 shows the temporal relationships of the clinical and hormonal indicators to the derived fertile period in the one conceptional cycle which occurred.

The calendar calculation S-19, the day of E_1-3-G rise and the day of the E_1-3-G/Pd-3α-G ratio all occurred outside the derived fertile period. In this cycle no mucus appeared until day -4, i.e. within the derived fertile period.

The end of the fertile period was correctly determined by both the basal body temperature and peak mucus indicators.

Sexual intercourse on day -5 resulted in a pregnancy which went to term.

This woman ignored the calendar calculations S-19 and relied solely on the first appearance of mucus to detect the beginning of the fertile period. Day -5 being a dry day was infertile and available for sexual intercourse. Had the calendar calculation S-19 been used to indicate the beginning of the fertile period and sexual intercourse discontinued after day -7 it is reasonable to expect that the pregnancy might not have occurred.

CONCLUSION

In this study, the most reliable clinical indicator to detect the beginning of the derived fertile period was the calendar calculation S-19. Mucus was not always

8

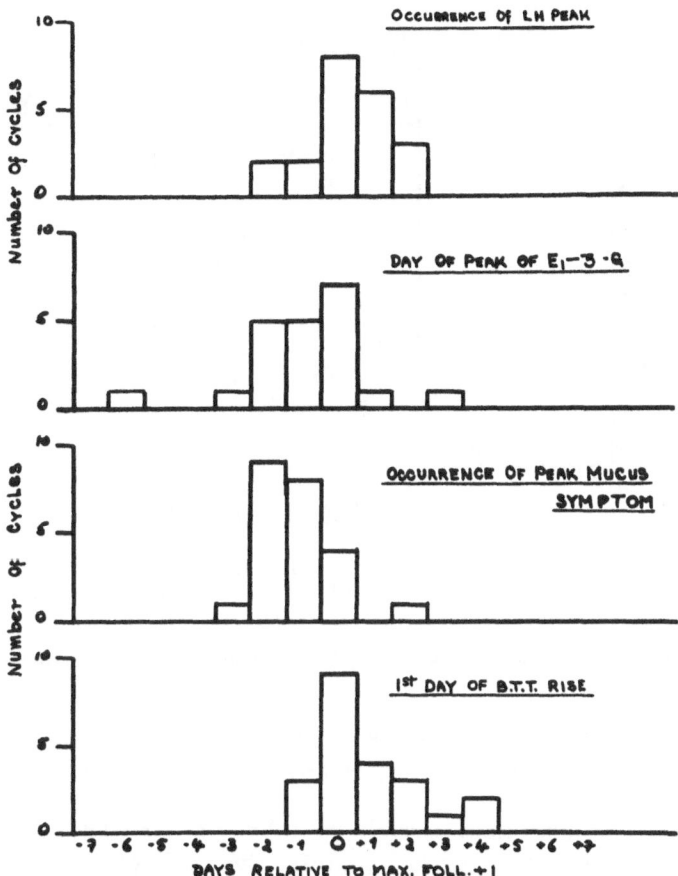

INDICATORS OF THE FERTILE PERIOD

Figure 4 Temporal relationship of the clinical and chemical indicators to the end of the derived fertile time

present sufficiently early enough to detect the first fertile day when one wished to avoid a pregnancy.

The current teaching of the double-check methodology – S-19 or the first appearance of mucus, whichever comes first – to detect the *beginning of the fertile period* appears to offer the most reliable combination of indicators at the present moment[4]. For this part of the cycle the chemical indicators E_1-3-G and E_1-3-G/Pd-3α-G ratio do not, in their present form, offer any increased reliability.

The *end of the fertile period* can be identified with reasonable accuracy by both the basal body temperature and the peak mucus symptom, although in a minute number of cycles one or other of these may fall within the fertile period. Using the double-check the morning of the third day after

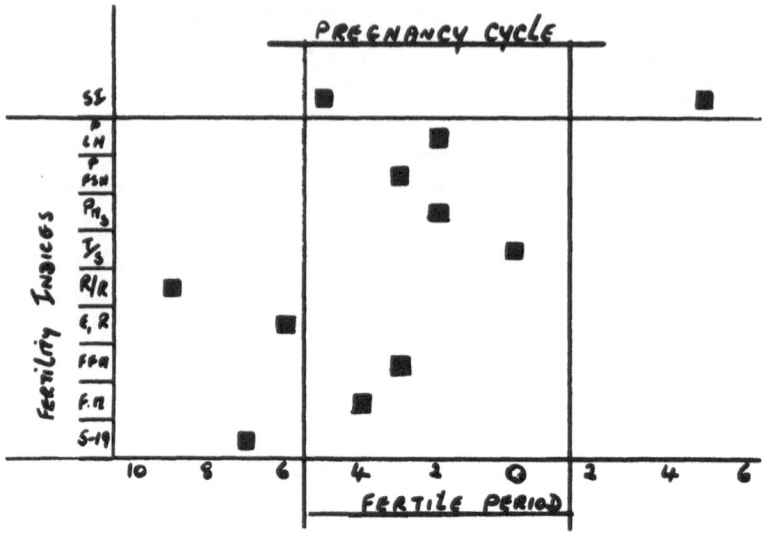

S.I. = Sexual intercourse; PLH = Peak LH; PFSH = Peak FSH; PMS = Peak mucus sympton; T/S = Temperature shift; R/R = Ratio rise; $E_1R = E_1$-3-G rise; FFM = First fertile mucus; FM = First mucus; Calender calculations.

Figure 5   Temporal relationships of clinical and chemical indicators to the derived fertile time

the temperature shift or the evening of the fourth day after the peak mucus symptom, whichever comes last – one can expect very few unplanned pregnancies.

In order to establish more securely the validity of these NFP parameters a larger study is necessary. For such a prospective study of the probability of conception at both ends of the presumed fertile time, this preliminary communication could serve as a protocol model.

ACKNOWLEDGEMENTS

We are indebted to the Clinical Research Centre, Northwick Park Hospital, Watford Road, Harrow, Middlesex, who helped financially with transport of the women to the Ultrasound Clinic, to our NFP tutors who helped recruit the women, and finally our sincere thanks go to the patients who volunteered for the study.

References

1. Kerin, J. F., Edmonds, D. K., Warnes, G. M., Cox, L. W., Seamark, R. F., Matthews, C. D., Young, G. B. and Baird, D. T. (1981). Morphological and functional relations of graafian follicle growth to ovulation in which women using ultrasonic, laporoscopic and biochemical measurements. *Br. J. Obstet. Gynaecol.*, **88**, 81–90

2. Collins, W. P., Collins, P. O., Kilpatrick, M. J., Manning, P. A., Pike, J. and Tyler, J. P. P. (1979). The concentration of oestrone-3-glucuronide, LH and pregnanediol-3α-glucuronide as indices of ovarian function. *Acta Endocrinol. (kβH).*, **93**, 123
3. Lynch, S. S. and Shirley, A. (1975). Productions of specific antisera to follicle stimulating hormone and other hormones. *J. Endocrinol.*, **65**, 127
4. W.H.O. Family Fertility Education Resource Package (1983). The Sympto-thermal module.

2
Natural family planning and hormonal assays in Japan

H. HONJO, J. YASUDA, J. KITAWAKI, T. KASEKI, A. ZIMMERMAN,
T. NAMBARA AND H. OKADA

INTRODUCTION

The ovulation method of natural family planning[1] was introduced as a natural and effective method to Japanese women in 1975. Hormonal features, including a conjugated oestrogen, were investigated in urine and serum from women who were infertile and using the ovulation method.

SUBJECTS AND METHODS

Subjects

Early morning urine samples every day throughout the menstrual cycle and serum samples (drawn between 1000 h and 1300 h) every day around the ovulation period were collected in four infertile women (29–32 years old), who were outpatients at the Kaseki Hospital, Nagoya, Japan and using the ovulation method of natural family planning as one of indicators of knowing the time of ovulation. Each woman monitored her own sequence of changes in the quality of cervical mucus and basal body temperature throughout the menstrual cycle. The serum and urinary samples were stored at $-20°C$ until analysed.

Reagents

$[6,7-^3H]$oestradiol-17-glucosiduronate (E_2-17-G) (45.6 Ci/mmol) was purchased from New England Nuclear (Boston, MA, USA). All other steroids were purchased from Sigma Chemical Co. (St. Louis, MO, USA). Organic solvents and chemicals were of analytical grade.

13

Urinary RIA of E_2-17-G

The antiserum used was obtained from a rabbit immunized with E_2-17-G-bovine serum albumin (BSA) conjugate in which the hapten was linked to the carrier protein through the C-2 position. The antibody had a high specificity for E_2-17-G. The urinary RIA of E_2-17-G was performed according to the method described elsewhere[2].

Serum E_2, LH and urinary LH

Serum E_2 was measured with oestradiol radioimmunoassay kit (CEA-IRE-SORIN, France) and LH with LH-RIA kit (Daiichi Radioisotope laboratories Ltd., Tokyo, Japan). Urinary LH was measured with a HCG-HAR kit (Mochida pharmaceutical Ltd., Tokyo, Japan).

RESULTS

Table 1 summarizes the results. A vaginal sensation of wetness was observed 12–3 days earlier than the peak day of urinary LH. The mucus became lubricative 3 days earlier to 1 day later than the day of peak urinary LH, namely 2 days earlier to 2 days later than the day of peak serum oestradiol. The urinary E_2-17-G peak appeared 3–1 day earlier than the urinary LH peak day, and the level of these preovulatory peaks were 15.8–29.6 $\mu g/l$.

Table 1 Time relationship between beginning of sensation of wetness (W), changing to lubricative (L), urinary E_2-17-G peak and urinary LH peak

day case	−13	−12	−11	−10	−9	−8	−7	−6	−5	−4	−3	−2	−1	LH peak day	+1
M.K.											W E_2-17-G-P				L
T.K.											W E_2-17-G-P		L		
H.S.					W						L	E_2-17-G-P			
Y.T.	W										L		E_2-17-G-P		

DISCUSSION

A prospective multicentre trial of the ovulation method was performed by WHO and the results were reported[1] in 1981.

The pregnancy rate was good, only 2.8 pregnancies per 100 women years in effectiveness phase. But the mean number of days of abstinence required was 15.4. Also in the present study with four cycles with ovulations, somewhat long fertile periods (maximum, 12 + 4 days after LH peak = 16 days) were visible. It may be somewhat long.

E_2-17-G is specific for human. Preovulatory E_2-17-G peaks were reported[3].

14

In the present study with the different antibody antiserum to E$_2$-17-G-[C-2]-BSA), urinary peak of E$_2$-17-G appeared 3–1 day earlier than the urinary LH peak day. The measurement of E$_2$-17-G may predict more exactly than the sensation of wetness in the ovulation method. The ovulation method of natural family planning plus biochemical indicators would be more practical to control fertility and also to treat infertility.

ACKNOWLEDGEMENTS

This study was supported by WHO (project Number 80063, 1981, Number 81909H, 1982) and Grant-in-Aid for Scientific Research, Japan (project Number 56480280, 1981, 1982).

References

1. World Health Organization, Task Force on Methods for the Determination of the Fertile Period, Special Programme of Research, Development and Research Training in Human Reproduction: A prospective multicentre trial of the ovulation method of natural family planning. II. The effectiveness phase (1981). *Fertil. Steril.*, **36**, 591
2. Numazawa, M., Tanaka, T. and Nambara, T. (1979). Determination of estrogen ring D glucuronides in pregnancy plasma by direct radioimmunoassay without hydrolysis. *Clin. Chim. Acta*, **91**, 169
3. Branch, C. M., Collins, P. O. and Collins, W. P. (1982). Ovulation prediction: Changes in the concentrations of urinary estrone-3-glucuronide, estradiol-17 beta-glucuronide and estriol-16 alpha-glucuronide during conceptional cycles. *J. Steroid Biochem.*, **16**, 345

3
Billings natural FP method: correlation of subjective signs with ovulation and cervical mucus quality

J. J. ETCHEPAREBORDA, L. VIDELA, S. BORTOLUSSI AND E. KESSERÜ

INTRODUCTION

Amongst the different methods of 'natural' family planning, the vulvar humidity or 'moistness' appraisal introduced by Billings[1], seems to represent an advance, since it offers an additional – through subjective – means of predicting fertile days. The aim of the present study was not to search for the clinical efficacy of the Billings method, but to correlate the subjective feelings, reported by the women, with actual cervical mucus quality, e.g. penetrability, as well as the actual time of ovulation.

SUBJECTS

Fifty-one highly motivated volunteers with proven fertility, were studied through 62 ovulatory cycles. They were taught and trained to record, day by day, the degree of vulvar humidity sensation according to a conventional scale that ranged from 'no humidity' ($-$) up to 'maximal humidity' ($+ + +$). Patients were also asked to record their basal body temperatures.

METHODS

The methodology followed in each cycle is summarized in Figure 1. Cervical mucus quality was assessed daily or interdaily by quantifying spinnbarkeit (cm) and ferning (%) by means of the crystallometer[2]. Simultaneously, serial colpocytograms were made. As soon as mucus plus colpocytology indicated the

17

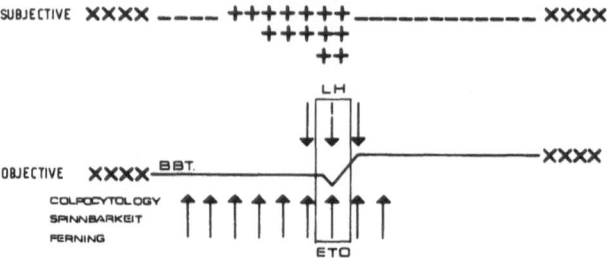

Figure 1 Methods . Scheme of one cycle. 'Subjective': humidity degree reported by the women. 'Objective': assessment of cervical mucus and ovulation patterns. XXXX: menstrual days, ETO: estimated time of ovulation

imminence of the ovulatory phase of the cycle, the estimated time of ovulation (ETO) was pinpointed by daily LH measurement. All the described parameters were matched with the daily humidity degree reported by the women.

RESULTS

The relation of subjective humidity with cervical mucus quality is shown in Figure 2 (spinnbarkeit) and Figure 3 (crystallization). The distributions of both parameters showed a relationship to humidity degree with high statistical significance.

The ETO was also closely related with the vulvar humidity, taking into account the 'peak days', as described by Billings[1] (i.e. the last day of maximal

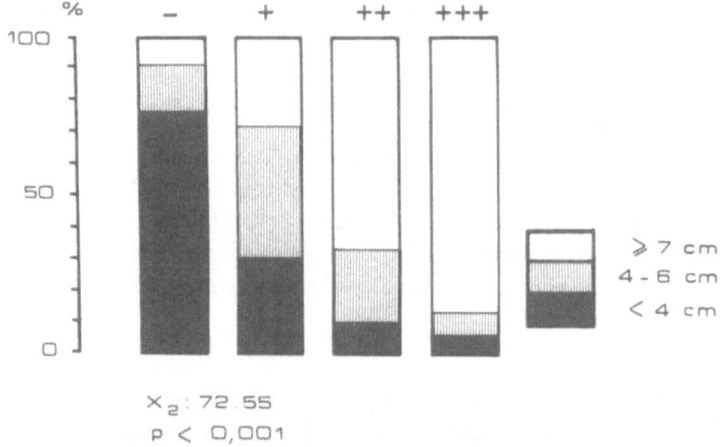

Figure 2 Vulvar humidity degree vs. cervical mucus spinnbarkeit. Columns represent the different humidity degrees and the simultaneous distribution of spinnbarkeit patterns

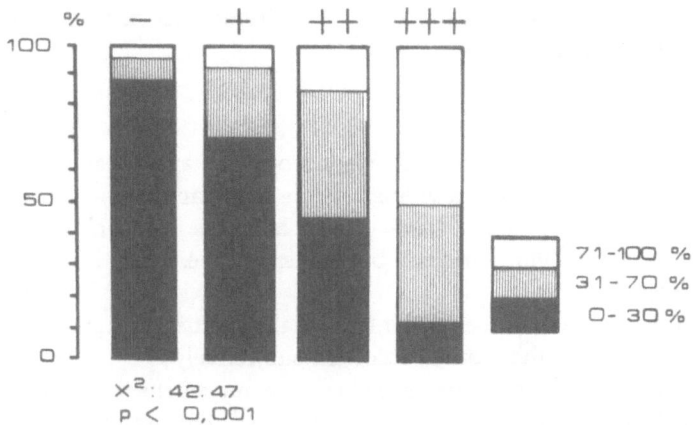

Figure 3 Vulvar humidity degree vs. cervical mucus ferning. Columns represent the different humidity degrees and the simultaneous distribution of ferning patterns expressed in per cent of crystallization of the mucus sample

humidity); 87% of these peak days were found at ETO day -2, -1, 0 and $+1$. In 91% of the cycles the humid days started on ETO day -5 and ended on ETO day $+1$. Statistical analysis (Figure 4) showed that the proportions of

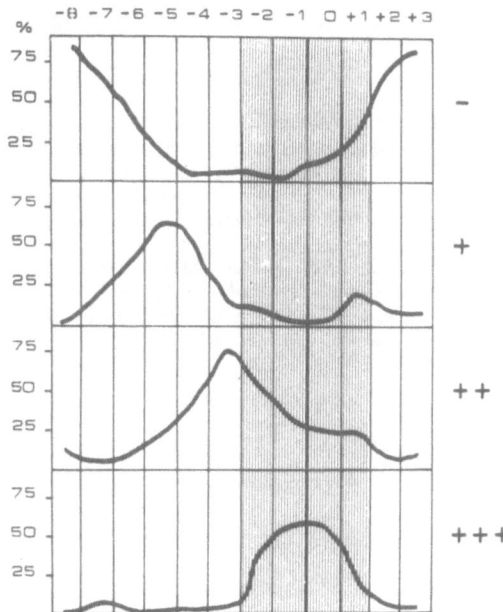

Figure 4 Proportional incidence of the different humidity degrees in comparison with ETO

different humidity degrees (+ to + + +) yielded successive waves moving towards ETO day '0'.

DISCUSSION

The patients dealt with in our study were motivated and collaborative enough as to have no problems in providing reliable self-examination data. This may not apply to every FP user. However, our aim was not to check the clinical applicability of the Billings method but rather to investigate the consistency of its physiological bases.

Under this approach the cervical mucus quality patterns did show a very close relationship to what the women recorded subjectively.

On the other hand the dependence of cervical mucus rheology with its ability to be penetrated by spermatozoa is well known[3]. For example, in a previous study we have already demonstrated that with less than 30% crystallization no sperm entrance into the uterine cavity is possible[2]; in the present study this was the case in 88% of women reporting no humidity sensation.

The relationship of the Billings method with actual cervical mucus quality has been corroborated by others[4]. Concerning the correlation of the vulvar humidity with the ETO our results appeared quite consistent with other reports[5].

In conclusion the Billings method, if correctly taught and applied, is based on a sound physiological basis, and is suitable for natural family planning.

References

1. Billings, J. J. (1964). *The Ovulation Method*. (Melbourne: Advocate Press)
2. Kesserü, E. (1972). A Simple Method for Measuring Crystallization of the Cervical Mucus and its Application in Human Sperm Migration. *Int. J. Fertil.*, **17**, 201
3. Kesserü, E. (1973). Assessment of the Rheology of Cervical Mucus. In Elstein, M., Moghissi, K. S. and Borth, R. (eds.) *Cervical Mucus in Human Reproduction*. pp. 45–57 (Copenhagen: Scriptor)
4. Hilgers, T. W. and Prebil, A. M. (1979). The Ovulation Method – Vulvar Observations as an Index of Fertility/Infertility. *Obstet. Gynecol.*, **53**, 12
5. Hilgers, T. W., Abraham, G. E. and Cavanagh, D. (1978). NFP. I The Peak Symptom and Estimated Time of Ovulation. *Obstet. Gynecol.*, **52**, 575

4
Clinical evaluation of endocrine profile by BBT records in dysovulatory infertility

B. N. CHAKRAVARTY AND S. CHATTOPADHYAY

INTRODUCTION

It is known that the Basal Body Temperature (BBT) chart indicates ovulatory status and perhaps in addition, reflects the extent of functional adequacy of the corpus luteum in the luteal phase. But it appeared from our study that almost the entire reproductive endocrine profile, normal or abnormal, can be, to a large extent, imaged in the BBT if this is correctly recorded and judiciously interpreted.

THERMOGENIC HORMONES

It is well known that progesterone has a thermogenic action which is mediated through the central nervous system[3]; androgens like progesterone have a similar effect. Hence the rise in temperature during the menstrual cycle is due to the appearance of the increased blood concentrations of these hormones.

With advancing knowledge in reproductive endocrinology over the last few years various drugs are being used for inducing ovulation and luteal support in dysovulatory infertility. The term 'dysovulatory' includes infertility associated with non-ovulation, infrequent or oligo ovulation, corpus luteum inadequacy and a discordant follicular phase. The indication and use of a specific drug is often based on the results of radioimmunoassay, and if facilities do not exist the drugs are used empirically accepting a 'trial and error' basis. Even if facilities are available, daily sampling of blood or urine is inconvenient to the patient, costly in laboratory charges and the hormonal profile that is obtained, while important in research studies, usually offers little value in clinical management. From the practical point of view, it may not be possible to assess daily the hormonal status in an infertile woman by radio-immuno-assay.

Recording BBT does not involve any cost; and at the same time gives an overview of the ovulatory status and endocrine profile during the period she is under treatment with ovulation inducing drugs.

SUBJECTS

Over the last 10 years each infertile woman attending our clinic has been asked to record her BBT while following a programme of other investigations for infertility. During this period (January 1973–December 1982) 3462 infertile women attended our clinic, and systematic recording of relevant data including the BBT chart have been analysed in all cases. 1521 had dysovulatory infertility giving an incidence of 43.93%. The diagnosis of dysovulatory infertility was based primarily on BBT patterns supplemented in some cases by endometrial biopsy and vaginal cytology. The interpretation of BBT patterns was subsequently correlated in 112 cases by estimation of hormones using blood and urine samples (Table 1).

Table 1 Correlation between abnormal BBT and endocrine profile (estimated from blood or urine)

Number of cases investigated endocrinologically	112
BBT pattern substantiated by endocrine assay	70
Inconclusive by endocrine assay	42

RECORDING BBT

The temperature is taken in the morning immediately on awakening and before arising. Reading and recording the temperature immediately after it is taken is not necessary. Attempting to read the thermometer while not yet fully awake may contribute not only to a lack of precision, but also to arousing antagonism against the method. The advantage of recording the temperature at leisure later in the day outweighs any slight error due to very minor contraction of the mercury column.

The thermometer of choice is especially designed for recording basal temperature, has an expanded scale over a limited range and an easily visualized mercury column, but for an intelligent patient an ordinary thermometer is equally good.

It is preferable to record the temperature at approximately the same time each day. When a significant variation in waking time occurs (more than one hour) fluctuations due to the diurnal variations in basal temperature may complicate the temperature chart record[1]. Such episodes of variable waking time (more than one hour) occur very infrequently in a month. However, a method for correcting temperatures for differing waking times has been proposed recently by Royston et al.[2].

The temperature can be taken orally, vaginally or rectally. Oral temperatures are slightly lower than vaginal or rectal, but the biphasic pattern of the ovulatory cycle is similar for all three records. In our series, oral temperature has been recorded.

RESULTS

Types of BBT evaluated and their interpretations

In our study, it has been observed that there could be basically six types of BBT charts (Table 2).

Table 2   Types of BBT in different endocrine profile

Types of BBT			Endocrine Profile
Biphasic			normal ovulatory
	Elevated monophasic		androgenic PCO
			hyperprolactinaemia
			with hyperadrenalism
Monophasic		Flat	hypothyroidism
			hypogonad. hypogonadism
			POF
			hyperprolactinaemia
	Low monophasic	Discordant	without hyperadrenalism
Discordant throughout			PCO (oestrogenic)
Short luteal			insufficient progesterone
Discordant luteal			fluctuating progesterone
Discordant follicular			early phase of hyperactive adrenal (initial phase of androgenic PCO)

Biphasic (Indicating normal ovulatory pattern)

The shift or rise in BBT which occurs at the time of ovulation is usually of the order of 0.3 °F to 0.5 °F. In a study carried out by Marshall[4] only 10% of cycles showed a thermal dip preceding the temperature rise and concluded that the rise could be one of three types. An acute rise with an elevation of at least 0.4 °F (0.2 °C) between two consecutive days, a slow gradual rise usually over 3–5 days but occasionally longer, or a step-like rise. Temperature charts illustrating three types of shifts are shown in Figures 1a, 1b and 1c.

23

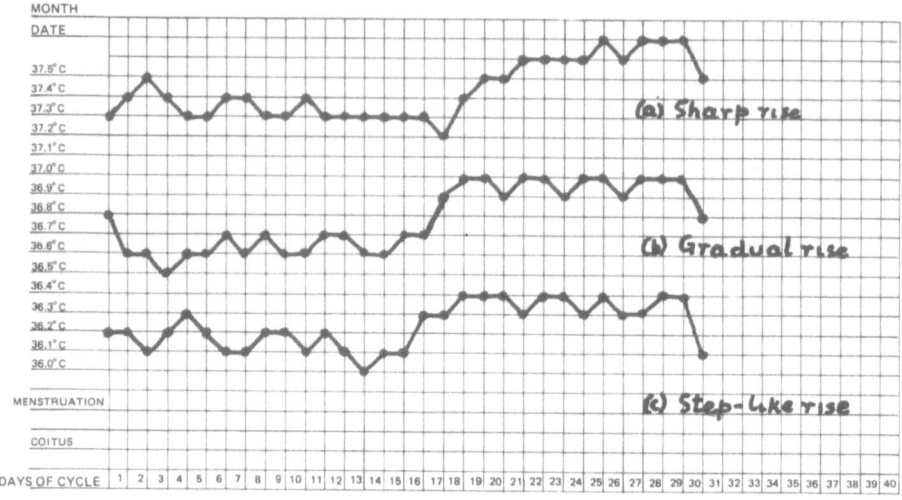

Figure 1(a), (b) & (c) BBT – Normal ovulatory

Monophasic

All women having monophasic BBT are non-ovulatory, and hence have low or absent progesterone levels. The normal temperature varies between 96.4–98.4 °F. Presuming 97.4–97.6 °F as the base line, monophasic types may be one of the following varieties.

(1) Elevated monophasic

The basal body temperature persistently remains above 97.8 °F throughout the cycle (Figure 2). Because of the absence or low levels of progesterone, it may be presumed that elevated monophasic BBT is the effect of an elevated level of androgen in the circulation. We have observed such types of persistent elevation in androgenic polycystic ovarian disease, and in very few cases of hyperprolactinaemia. It has been documented that excess adrenal androgen in response to ACTH stimulation may cause hyperovarianism and other manifestations of PCO[5]. It has also been shown that patients with hyperprolactinaemia may have elevated ketosteroids and hirsutism[6].

We have observed that the majority of persistently elevated BBTs was associated with androgenic PCO, the prolactin level remaining normal. In a small number of cases, we have found an elevated BBT with high rise in the level of pro-lactin. In hyperolactinaemia, the shift of BBT from low monophasic variety to elevated monophasic type did occur over a period of months or years, thereby indicating that in the initial phase of hyperprolactinaemia the temperature

24

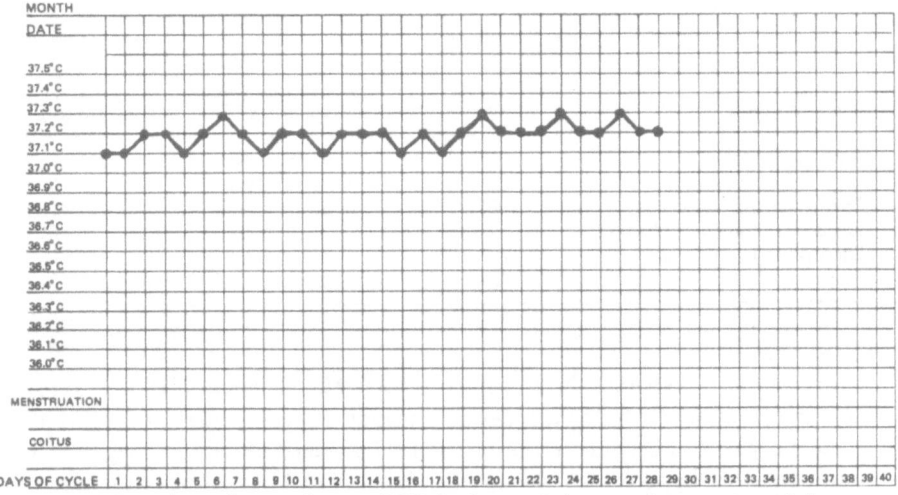

Figure 2 BBT – elevated monophasic – PCO (androgenic), hyperprolactinaemia with hyperadrenalism

remains low monophasic (see below); and if the state of hyperprolactinaemia continues, this will bring about hyperadrenalism and hyperovarianism (similar to androgenic PCO) leading to an elevated monophasic BBT pattern.

A clinical differentiation between hyperprolactinaemia and androgenic PCO resulting in elevated BBT has been observed during the course of treatment with dexamethasone. In cases of androgenic PCO, following induction with dexamethasone, the cervical mucus becomes abundant with maximum threadability

Table 3 Abnormal BBT pattern substantiated by endocrine assay (70 cases)

Types of abnormal BBT	No. of cases investigated endocrinologically		Endocrine profile	
		16	FSH LH	marked elevation (POF)
Low flat monophasic	30	4	FSH LH	modest reduction (hypogonad. hypogonadism)
		10	TSH	elevated
Low discordant monophasic	27		prolactin	elevated
Elevated monophasic	13	8	cortisol 17-ketosteroid	elevated
		5	prolactin	elevated

25

Table 4 Clinical response to ovulation inducing and luteal phase supporting drugs in women with abnormal BBT pattern (1521 cases)

Types of abnormal BBT	No. of cases	Correction of BBT pattern following treatment	Conception
Low monophasic	543	321 (59.1%)	105 (32.7%)
Elevated monophasic	222	102 (45.9%)	42 (41.1%)
Discordant throughout	104	57 (54.8%)	12 (21.1%)
Discordant follicular phase	33	11 (33.3%)	2 (18.1%)
Discordant luteal phase	290	196 (67.6%)	61 (31.1%)
Short luteal	329	205 (62.3%)	93 (45.3%)

(spinnbarkeit). Whereas in hyperprolactinaemic elevated BBT the cervical changes in midcycle following dexamethasone induction remains negative.

Our concept of elevated monophasic BBT associated with androgenic PCO and persistent hyperprolactinaemia has been corroborated by radioimmunoassay in 13 cases and therapeutic trial with dexamethasone in 222 cases (Tables 3 and 4).

(2) Low monophasic

This type of BBT persistently remaining below 97.6 °F may be due to (a) hypogonadotrophic hypogonadism, (b) hypothyroidism, (c) early phase hyperprolactinaemia (unassociated with PCO) and (d) premature ovarian failure. There are two types of low monophasic BBT, reflecting different varieties of internal endocrine profile.

(a) *Persistently flat low monophasic BBT*

In hypogonadotrophic hypogonadism, hypothyroidism and premature ovarian failure, the BBT remains persistently low and flat (Figure 3). Apart from clinical features of menstrual deficiency and definite stigma of hypothyroidism, the differential diagnosis has to be corroborated by biochemical studies and radioimmunoassay techniques. Alternatively, failure to induce ovulation or menstruation either by clomiphene or by gonadotrophins leads to the suspicion of hypothyroidism or premature ovarian failure. Confirmation of the diagnosis of premature ovarian failure has to be made by ovarian biopsy.

(b) *Discordant low monophasic BBT*

The temperature remains well below 97.6 °F but there is day to day fluctuation ranging between 96 °F and 97.6 °F (Figure 4). This type of BBT is specific for the majority of cases of hyperprolactinaemia. This has been corroborated in our study by radio-immunoassay in 27 cases.

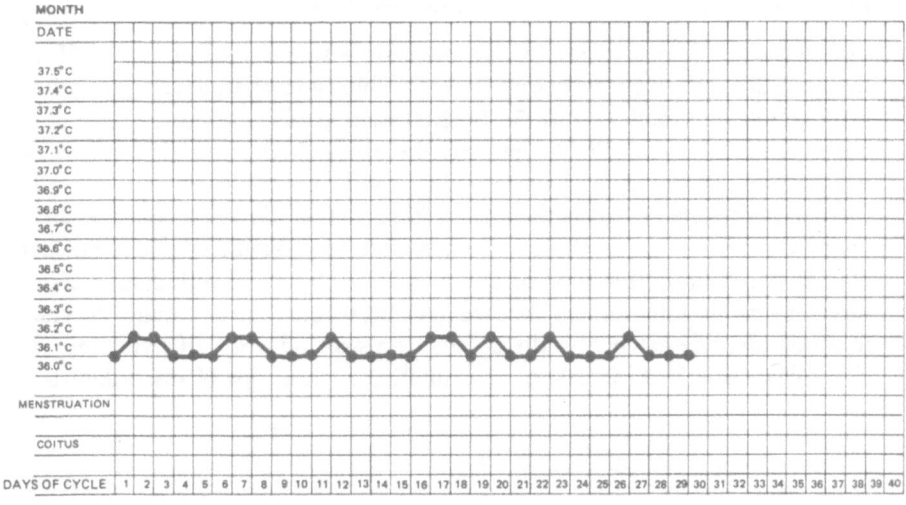

Figure 3 Low, flat monophasic (hypothyroidism; POF; hypogonad.; hypogonadism)

The small spikes in the temperature chart possibly indicate the beginning of adrenal stimulation, and if this state is allowed to continue for some time, an excess amount of adrenal androgen will be elaborated, the peripheral biologic effect of which will lead to a persistently elevated monophasic BBT.

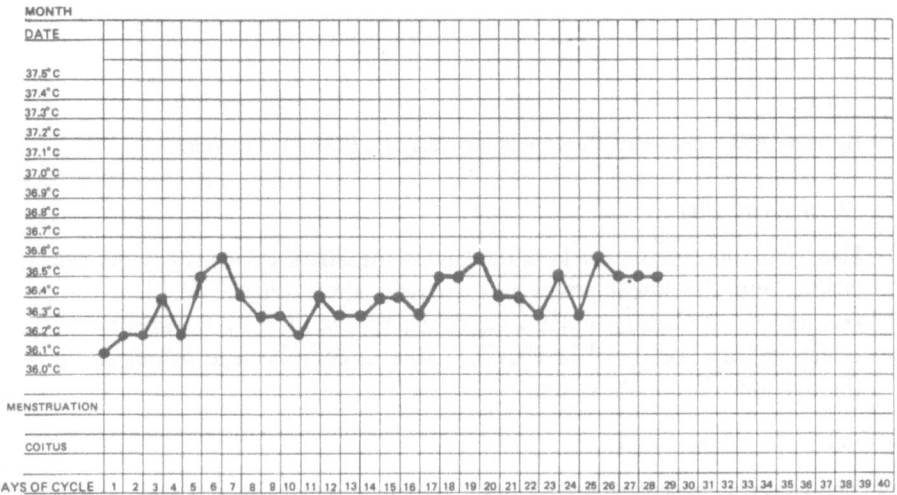

Figure 4 BBT – discordant low monophasic (hyperprolactinaemia (early phase))

Discordant throughout cycle, not specifically low

In this variety there is a day to day variation – sometimes below 97.8 °F and the next day this may go above 97.8 °F. This type of irrelevancy continues throughout the month (Figure 5). Such abnormal BBTs in our experience are observed in oestrogenic PCO where steroidogenesis in the ovary is defective due to an enzymatic defect. The sharp 'spikes' can be explained by nonaromatized ovarian androgens, whereas the regular 'dips' in the BBT chart could be due to peripheral conversion of these androgens into oestrogens. We have not been able to corroborate this type of abnormal BBT by serial estimations of hormones by radioimmunoassay, but we have been able to substantiate our views, to a considerable extent, by therapeutic trials of induction of ovulation with clomiphene and HCG in 104 cases exhibiting such a type of discordant BBT.

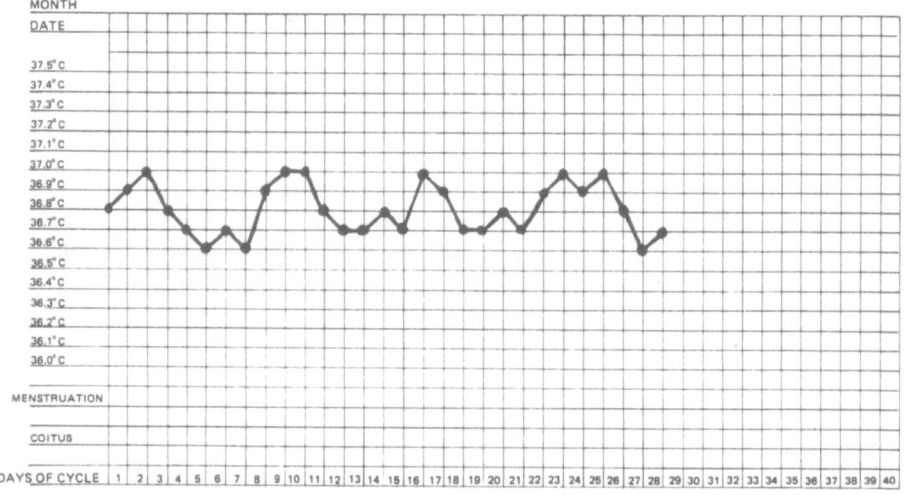

Figure 5   BBT – discordant throughout (anovulatory, PCO – oestrogenic)

Short luteal BBT

Here ovulation occurs at a later date in the menstrual cycle usually between day 20–24, and the luteal phase is extremely short (Figure 6). The treatment consists of antedating ovulation and helping nidation by luteal support (progesterone, allyl oestrinol or HCG). This was corroborated in our study by a therapeutic trial in 329 cases.

Discordant luteal BBT

This is a type of ovulatory BBT but is another variety of inadequacy of the luteal phase (Figure 7); because of fluctuations in the blood concentration of

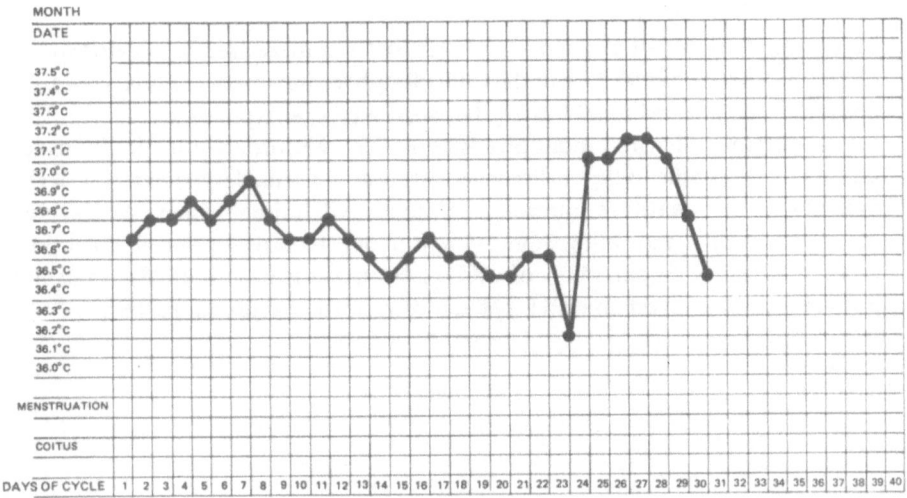

Figure 6 BBT – short luteal (ovulatory, inadequate luteal)

progesterone there are frequent temperature dips in the luteal phase. This can be corrected only by luteal support with luteotrophic drugs. In the present series, correction was achieved in 196 out of 290 cases.

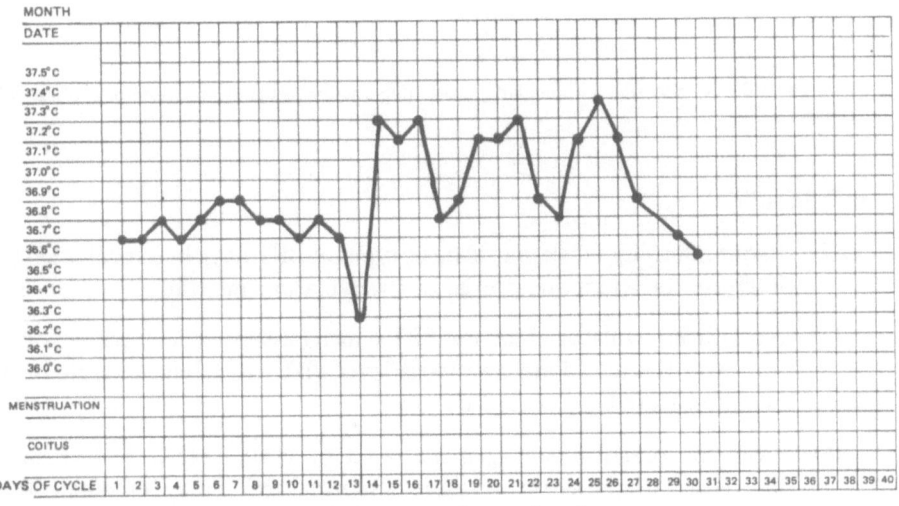

Figure 7 BBT – discordant luteal (ovulatory, inadequate luteal)

Discordant follicular phase BBT

This is also a variety of ovulatory biphasic BBT but there are few isolated spikes of temperature above 97.6 °F in the follicular phase (Figure 8). This type of BBT appears to be a transitional variety between a typical biphasic ovulatory BBT and a sustained elevated monophasic type. The discordancy in the follicular phase is perhaps due to the earlier manifestation of adrenal hyperactivity. If the patient remains infertile for quite some time she will ultimately have an elevated monophasic BBT indicating non-ovulation due to stress-induced polycystic ovarian disease[7]. Suppression of ACTH by dexamethasone in the follicular phase only may revert the BBT pattern to a normal biphasic pattern.

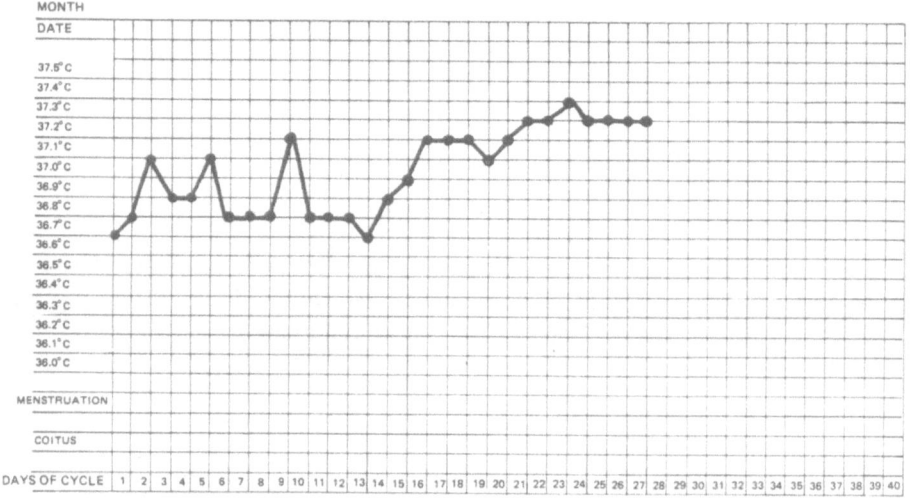

Figure 8 BBT – discordant follicular phase (hyperactive adrenal (premonitory phase of androgenic PCO))

SUMMARY

(1) In our infertility work up, six basic types of BBT have been evaluated to interpret the endocrine profile of dysovulatory infertility.

(2) Apart from ovulatory biphasic BBT which have been documented over the years, five additional new varieties of BBT which have attracted our attention have been recorded.

(3) From the practical management point of view, precise records and judicious interpretation of these abnormal BBT may eliminate the inconvenient and costly estimations of hormones from blood and urine.

(4) Besides detection of abnormal endocrine profiles in dysovulatory infertility, BBT records appear to be a useful clinical guide for follow-up after induction of ovulation with ovulation-inducing drugs.

References

1. Vollman, R. F. (1977). *The Menstrual Cycle Major Problems in Obstetrics and Gynaecology.* Vol. 7. (Philadelphia: W. B. Saunders)
2. Royston, J. P., Abrams, R. M., Higgins, M. P. and Flynn, A. (1980). *Br. J. Obstet. Gynaecol.*, **87**, 1123-7
3. Southan, S. L. and Gonzaga, F. P. (1965). *Am. J. Obstet and Gynaecol.*, **91**, 141-2
4. Marshall, J. (1963). *Br. Med. J.*, **1**, 102-4
5. Greenblatt, R. B. (1965). In R. B. Greenblatt (ed.) *The Hirsuit Female.* (Springfield: Charles C. Thomas)
6. Carter, J. N., Gomez, F. and Friesen, H. G. (1977). *Endocrine Causes of Menstrual Disorders.* Givens, J. R. (ed.) p. 115, (Chicago and London: Medical Year Book Publishers)
7. Chakravarty, B. N., Gun, K. M. and Mukherjee, S. (1980). *Indian J. Psychosom., Obstet. Gynaecol.*, **I**, 20-29

5
Fast procedures for serum LH with commercial reagents

J. H. SCHADE

INTRODUCTION

Accurate prediction of the time of ovulation is essential for the recovery of a mature oocyte for *in vitro* fertilization (IVF) and artificial insemination. Different commercial LH-kits were studied and optimized for short incubation times, and resulted in assays which can be completed within 90 minutes, and one within 45 minutes. The sensitivity of the 45 minute protocol is 2 IU/l (MRC 68/40).

MATERIALS AND METHODS

LH-kits were obtained from Byk-Mallinckrodt, Cis and Amersham. Sera were obtained from patients and stored at −20 °C. Calf serum (J. Rottier, Kloosterzande, Holland) was filtered through 0.4 μm and 0.22 μm filter (Sartorius, Germany). A low endogenous LH poolserum was obtained from hypogonadotropic females, this pool was also filtered. MRC 68/40 preparation was spiked on the calf serum pool and human LH pool serum in different amounts for recovery studies and for routine standard preparations. The standards were stored at −20 °C in small Eppendorf vials, and are stable for more than one year.

The Byk-Mallinckrodt kit was used as the reference method using the overnight protocol. Deming analysis were applied on data from the sequential incubations of the 30–30 minute protocol of all kits and 15–15 minute protocol for the Amersham kit. The B/F separation was achieved according to the kit insert protocol. The 15–15 minutes protocol of the Amersham kit uses

33

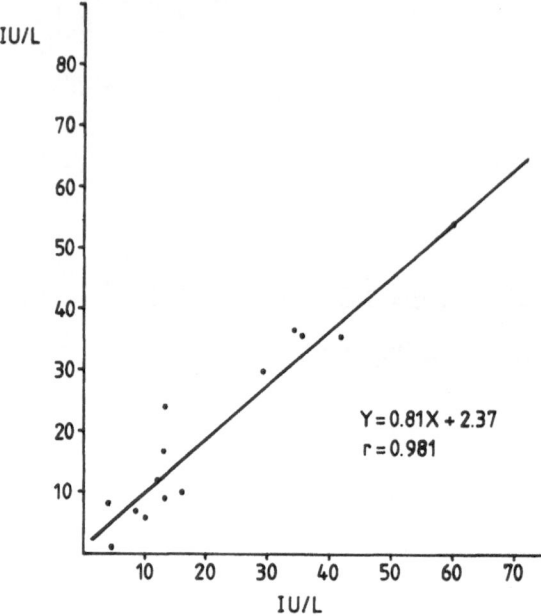

Figure 1 Scatterdiagram of the reference method (x) and short (30–30 minutes) Byk method using own kit standards

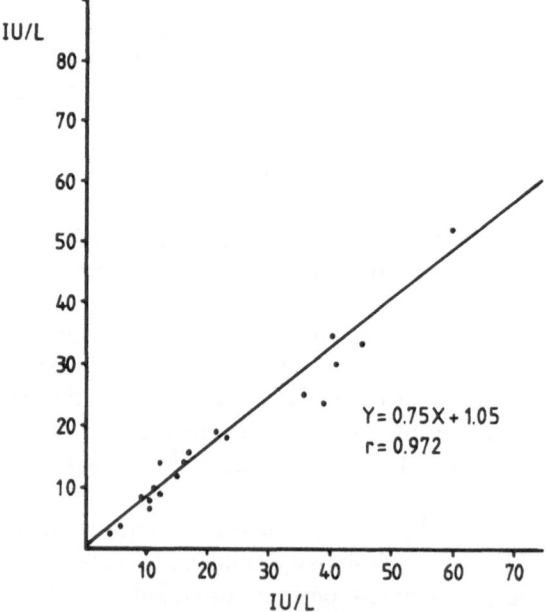

Figure 2 Scatterdiagram of the reference method (x) and short (30–30 minutes) Cis method using own kit standards

50 µl MRC standard in calf serum or human serum with the following concentrations: 12–22 and 44 IU/l combined with 50 µl anti-LH serum. After mixing on a SMI multivortex the plastic tubes are incubated for 15 minutes at 37 °C, 50 µl of ^{125}I-labelled LH is quickly added with a Hamilton repeating syringe, mixed and incubated for another 15 minutes at 37 °C, followed by 500 µl Amerlex second antibody and centrifuged after 10 minutes at 1500 g for 5 minutes. The supernatant is aspirated and the tubes are counted in a multi-well gamma counter (LKB, Finland).

RESULTS

The 30–30 minutes protocol of the three tested kits were compared to their own kit standards. The Byk method (Figure 1) showed good correlation, but is slightly imprecise in the 5–20 IU/l region. The Cis method (Figure 2) showed almost the same coefficient of correlation and was more precise in the low region.

The count rates obtained in both short 30–30 minutes protocol of Cis and Byk were much lower than obtained with the Amersham kit (Figure 3). These kits were not explored further for the 15–15 minutes protocol. The intra-assay coefficient of variation of the Amersham 15–15 minutes protocol (Figure 4, 5)

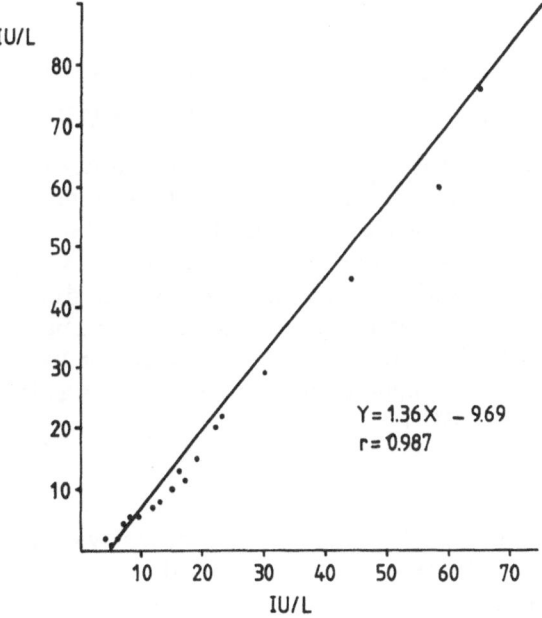

$$Y = 1.36X - 9.69$$
$$r = 0.987$$

Figure 3 Scatterdiagram of the reference method (x) and short (30–30 minutes) Amersham method using own kit standards

35

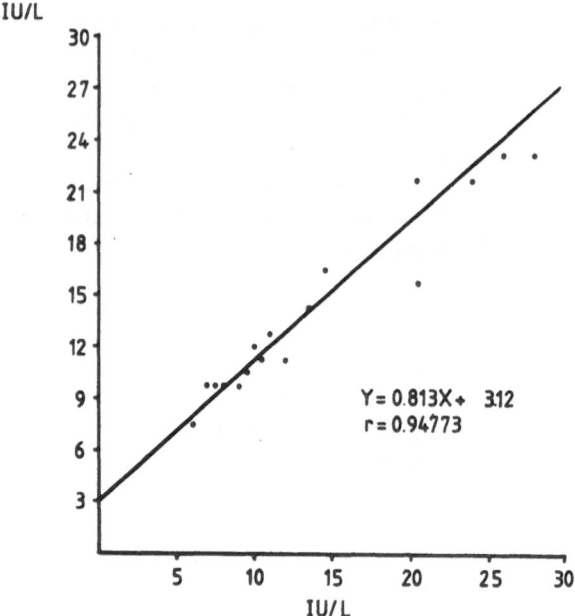

IU/L

Y = 0.813X + 3.12
r = 0.94773

IU/L

Figure 4 Scatterdiagram of the reference method (x) and short (15-15 minutes) Amersham method using MRC 68/40 in human serum

was measured in 12 samples at two different physiologically interesting levels:

$X = 9.05\,IU/l, \quad VC\,\% = 8.77 \quad$ and $\quad X = 25.11\,IU/l, \quad VC\,\% = 7.60$

MRC 68/40 spiked on the human pool serum and calf serum pool at four different levels 51, 26, 14 and 7 IU/l were analysed using the 3 point human serum standard curve. The recovery of the human pool standards was 103.5% an 101.8% for the calf serum standard. The calf serum pool showed an immuno-activity of 3.8 IU/l on the human serum standard curve. Sera with high endogenous LH showed good parallelism to calf and human serum standards. HCG (2nd IS) spiked on HCG free serum gave almost 100% cross-reactivity in the Amersham 15-15 minutes protocol. The HCG standard curve showed parallelism from 0-50 IU/l.

DISCUSSION

Until now fast LH assays were only possible for highly equipped laboratories, and the Amersham 15-15 minutes protocol is the fastest assay known today. Standards can be easily made up in calf serum or a human pool. The reaction of the label is so fast ($t\frac{1}{2}$ within 30 minutes) that the assay can be further optimized, but the sensitivity and precision over the whole curve is high enough.

In normal routine the three standard points and patient sample, diluted 1:1 and undiluted, is set up and the reagent costs are approximately 4 US dollars.

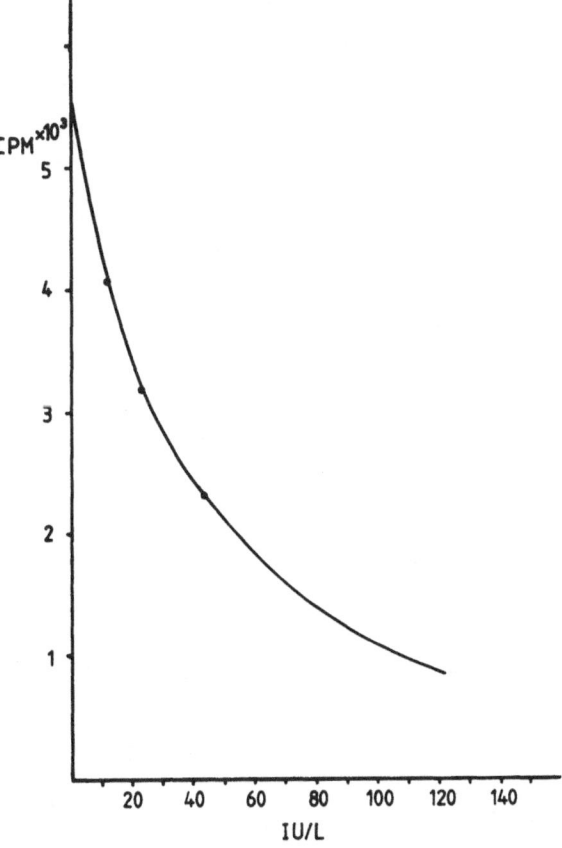

Figure 5 Standard curve of the (15–15 minutes) Amersham method with 3-point human standard curve

6

The optimization of an immunochemical test to locate the fertile period in women

L. E. M. SCHIPHORST, H. N. SALLAM, A. O. ADEKUNLE,
W. P. COLLINS AND J. P. ROYSTON

ABSTRACT

An immunochemical test, for predicting the limits of the fertile period and the time of maximum potential fertility in women, has been optimized by application to 118 menstrual cycles from apparently healthy women. The test is based upon changes in the concentration of oestrone-3-glucuronide (E_1-3-G) in daily samples of early morning urine (EMU). Two rises (R_1 and R_2) above a mean background level are determined by CUSUM analysis to give signals 72 hours and 24 hours before the time of the LH peak, or maximum follicular diameter (in 38 cycles). Subsequently, a peak level of E_1-3-G is identified and the end of potential fertility is calculated. The optimum number of days to determine the baseline, the appropriate reference levels to detect rise days 1 and 2, and the minimum number of days from the peak, have been studied in relation to the length of the derived fertile period. Under optimum conditions the test for the start and end of potential fertility was successful in 95% of cycles, and the mean length of the fertile period was 10.2 days (SD ± 2.7). The best test for maximum potential fertility gave a signal in 95% of cycles, with a mean time of 43 hours to the time of maximum follicular diameter. Eighty-two per cent of the signals occurred within the range + 48 hours to − 24 hours.

INTRODUCTION

The practice of family planning by periodic abstinence and the management of infertility imply the need for tests which determine accurately the limits of the fertile period (FP) and the time of maximum potential fertility (MPF) during each menstrual cycle. It may be deduced from a mathematical model of conception probabilities[1], which takes into account the life span of the gametes, that the start and end of the FP occur at approximately 72 hours before and 48 hours after ovulation. MPF (i.e. the time of maximum conception probability) occurs about 24 hours before ovulation. A practical immunochemical test[2], based on the measurement of oestrone-3-glucuronide (E_1-3-G) in daily samples of early morning urine (EMU), may be used for both the above clinical applications. The aim of the present study was to optimize the methods for (a) detecting a rise (R_1) in the pre-ovulatory concentration of E_1-3-G, to indicate the start of the FP; (b) determining a further rise (R_2) in E_1-3-G corresponding to the probable MPF; and (c) the identification of a peak value for E_1-3-G which is followed by the end of potential fertility in the current cycle.

EXPERIMENTAL PROCEDURE

The concentrations of E_1-3-G and LH were measured by radio-immunoassay in daily samples of EMU throughout 118 menstrual cycles (73 women). All subjects (aged 21–35 years) were in good health, and had a history of reasonably regular menstrual cycles (25–33 days). Thirty-eight women were scanned daily between 0800 and 1000 hours by ovarian ultrasonography to determine the time of maximum follicular diameter (MFD). Twelve women conceived during the period of study.

Previously, the E_1-3-G test identified the fertile period as the time between a sustained rise in the concentration (R_1) and the peak level plus 96 hours (4 days)[2]. The values for E_1-3-G in nmol/l were converted to $\log_e$ before analysis. A baseline was calculated as the mean value on days 1–6 for each cycle studied. A reference level for the cumulative sum (CUSUM) test (to determine R_1) was calculated as baseline plus 1 SD for the population (0.30 $\log_e$ units, k). The CUSUM test was performed by subtracting the reference level from each of the daily $\log_e$ values, and adding the result to the current CUSUM. The CUSUM was reset to zero if its value became negative. A statistically significant rise was recorded when the CUSUM reached a decision level, h, equal to 2 population SD units, i.e. 0.60. The day of the defined rise (R_1) was the day on which the data first exceeded the reference level in the run leading to the significant CUSUM (R_2 in the present study). The peak day for E_1-3-G was determined, prospectively, by starting with the R_1 plus 1 and selecting the day with a value that was followed by three consecutive lower amounts[2].

Definitions

Day 1 of the menstrual cycle was the first day of menstruation, i.e. the day starting after midnight on which there was a noticeable flow of blood through the vagina. The immunochemical test was usually started on day 2. The day of the LH peak was the day of the highest arithmetic value for the metabolite in EMU between days 5 and 25 of the menstrual cycle, and was determined retrospectively. The day of MFD was the day on which a follicle reached a mean diameter $\geqslant 18$ mm, and had reduced in size and acoustic density 24 hours later[3]. The probable FP for reference purposes was defined as: (a) the day of the LH peak -3 to the day of LH peak $+2$ inclusive, or (b) the day of MFD -2 to the day of MFD $+3$ inclusive. The duration of the derived fertile period was described in days (or 24 hour periods).

LIMITS OF THE FERTILE PERIOD

Effect of reference and decision levels

The effects of changing the CUSUM parameters k used to calculate the reference level, and h, the CUSUM decision level, are shown in Figure 1. It may be seen that as the values of k and h are increased, the test becomes arithmetically more stringent, thus the percentage of late signals goes up, while the number of false (i.e. early) signals for the end of the FP is reduced. The number of successful tests (i.e. those signals that circumscribe the fertile period) remains constant at about 80%. A value of 0.3 for k and 0.6 for h were selected for the evaluation of other variables.

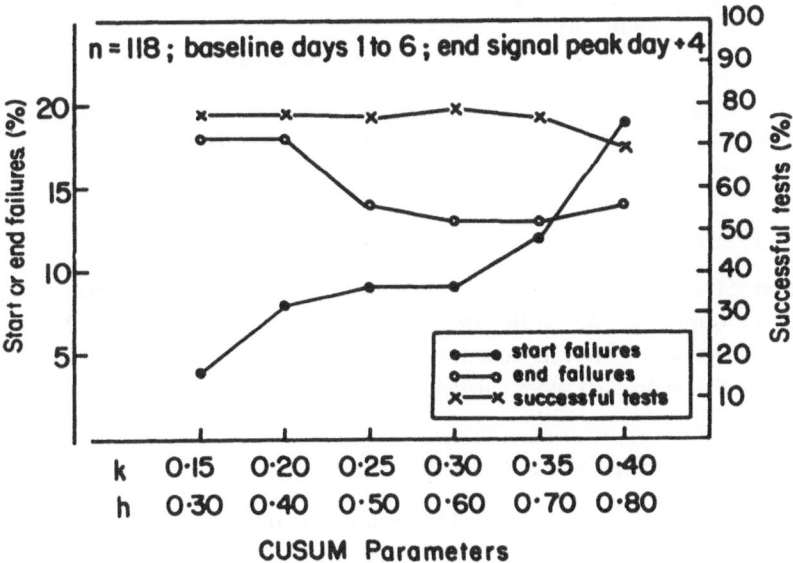

Figure 1 The effect of changing CUSUM values on the percentage of start and end failures and successful tests

Effect of peak-selecting algorithm

In practice, the end of potential fertility occurs at a varying time interval after the E_1-3-G peak. The effect of increasing this time interval on the overall success rate of the test is shown in Figure 2. There is a progressive increase in the mean length of the FP (from 8.5 to 13.3 days) while the success rate of the test is again reasonably constant at about 80%. The peak day +5 was selected as the best index for the end of the FP.

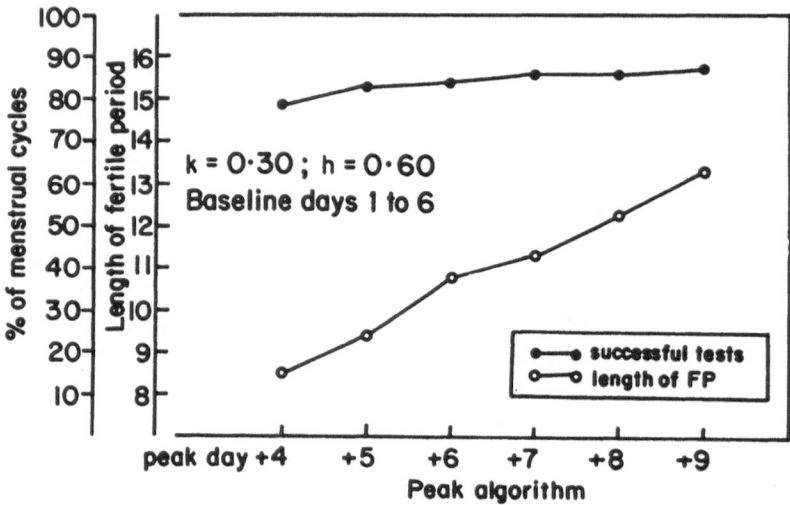

Figure 2 The effect of extending the time interval from the peak of E_1-3-G to identify the end of fertility on the percentage of successful tests and the length of the derived FP

Effect of baseline

Changing the number of days over which the baseline is calculated from 4 (days 2–5) to 6 (days 2–7) had little effect on the success rate of the test. The mean length of the derived fertile period, however, decreased from 10.9 to 10.4 days. Accordingly, days 2–6 were subsequently used as a compromise.

Effect of reference point for ovulation

The effect of using the day of the LH peak or the day of MFD as the reference point for ovulation (and hence the FP) on the success of the test is shown in Figure 3. The oestrone test is 95% effective when $k = 0.2$, $h = 0.4$ and MFD is used as the reference point.

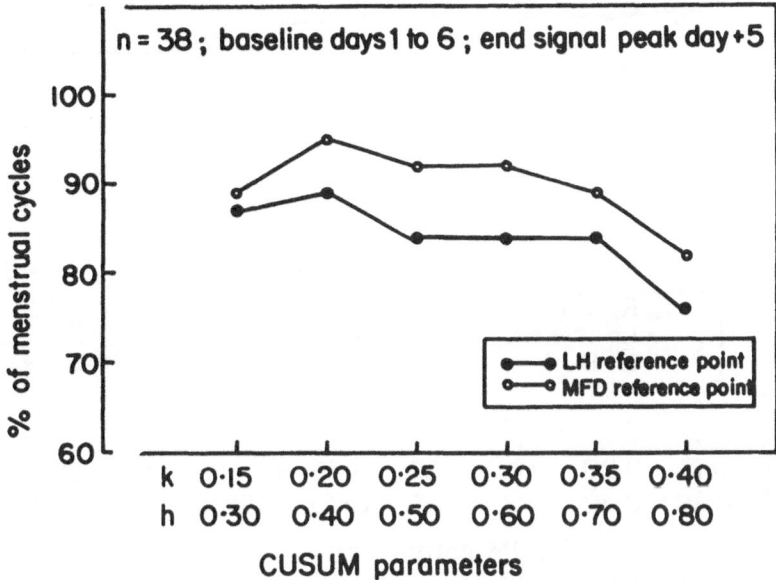

Figure 3 The effect of changing CUSUM values and the reference point for ovulation on the percentage of successful tests

PERIOD OF MAXIMUM FERTILITY

Effect of reference points and decision levels

The effect of increasing the CUSUM parameters k and h on the ability of the test to provide a signal for MFP in relation to the day of the LH peak or MFD is shown in Figure 4. When the values for k and h were 0.40 and 0.80 respectively, the test gave a signal during 95% of cycles. The mean time from the signal to the time of MFD was then 43 hours (SD 34). It was calculated that 82% of the signals occurred within the range of +48 hours to −24 hours, which probably represents the time of MPF.

CONCLUSIONS

Defined changes in the concentration of E_1-3-G in EMU were able to identify the limits of the FP and the probable time of MPF in approximately 95% of menstrual cycles with ultrasonic evidence of follicular rupture. The CUSUM-based algorithms appear to be robust, and the success rate of the test is not changed markedly by alterations of the baseline value, reference and decision levels, or time from the peak value. Further modifications of the algorithm, not described here, to restrict the day of the peak or to identify isolated high values have not improved the overall success rate. Accordingly, the results to date

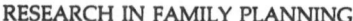

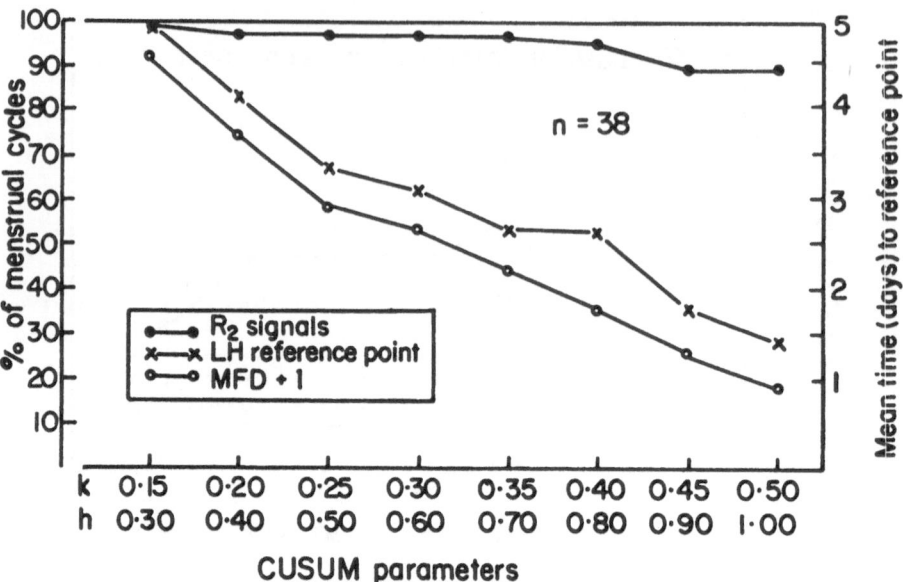

Figure 4 The effect of changing CUSUM values on the time intervals to two reference points for ovulation and the percentage of menstrual cycles with a signal

suggest that the test should be of value in the practice of reproductive medicine to help achieve or avoid a pregnancy. Attempts are in hand to simplify the assay procedure before the test is assessed in clinical trials.

ACKNOWLEDGEMENTS

The data storage, statistical and CUSUM analyses were performed with a Commodore 8032 microcomputer using the statistics package SPP (Supersoft Ltd., Harrow, UK).

References

1. Royston, J. P. (1982). Basal body temperature, ovulation and the risk of conception with special reference to the lifetimes of sperm and egg. *Biometrics*, **38**, 397–406
2. WHO Task Force on Methods for the Determination of the Fertile Period (1983): Temporal relationships between indices of the fertile period. *Fertil. Steril.*, **39**, 647–55
3. Queenan, J. T., O'Brien, G. D., Bains, L. M., Collins, P. O., Simpson, J., Collins, W. P. and Campbell, S. (1980). Ultrasound scanning of ovaries to detect ovulation in women. *Fertil. Steril.*, **34**, 99–105

7

The dual analyte assay for the detection of the fertile period in women

T. S. BAKER, R. J. HOLDSWORTH AND W. F. COULSON

ABSTRACT

The Dual Analyte assay (DAA), is described for assessing ovarian function in women. This test gives a colour signal as a function of the oestrone-3-glucuronide/pregnanediol-3-glucuronide (E/P) ratio in menstrual cycle urine. Since these are major metabolites of oestradiol and progesterone respectively, the DAA provides an index of follicular oestrogen as opposed to luteal phase oestrogen. (Signal due to luteal E being negated by high P.)

The DAA has been assessed for its ability to detect the period of maximum fertility (as located by ultrasound/urine LH) in 16 cycles by monitoring daily urine samples.

It was possible to select an absorbance threshold ($A_{570\,nm} = 0.37$) which was exceeded over one or more days during the pre-ovulatory phase of all 16 cycles. Absorbance values first exceeded the threshold between days -8 and 0 of each cycle; 81% of cycles demonstrating this rise between days -8 and -2. A final fall in absorbance values below the threshold was observed between days -2 and $+4$; 81% of cycles showing a fall over days $+1$ to $+3$. No 'false positive' values were observed before day -8 or after day $+4$.

The DAA provides a simple yes/no method for determining the period of maximum fertility and for giving warning of ovulation.

INTRODUCTION

The Dual Analyte assay produces a positive colour change in response to an increasing oestrone-3-glucuronide/pregnanediol-3-glucuronide (E_1-3-G/PD-3-G)

45

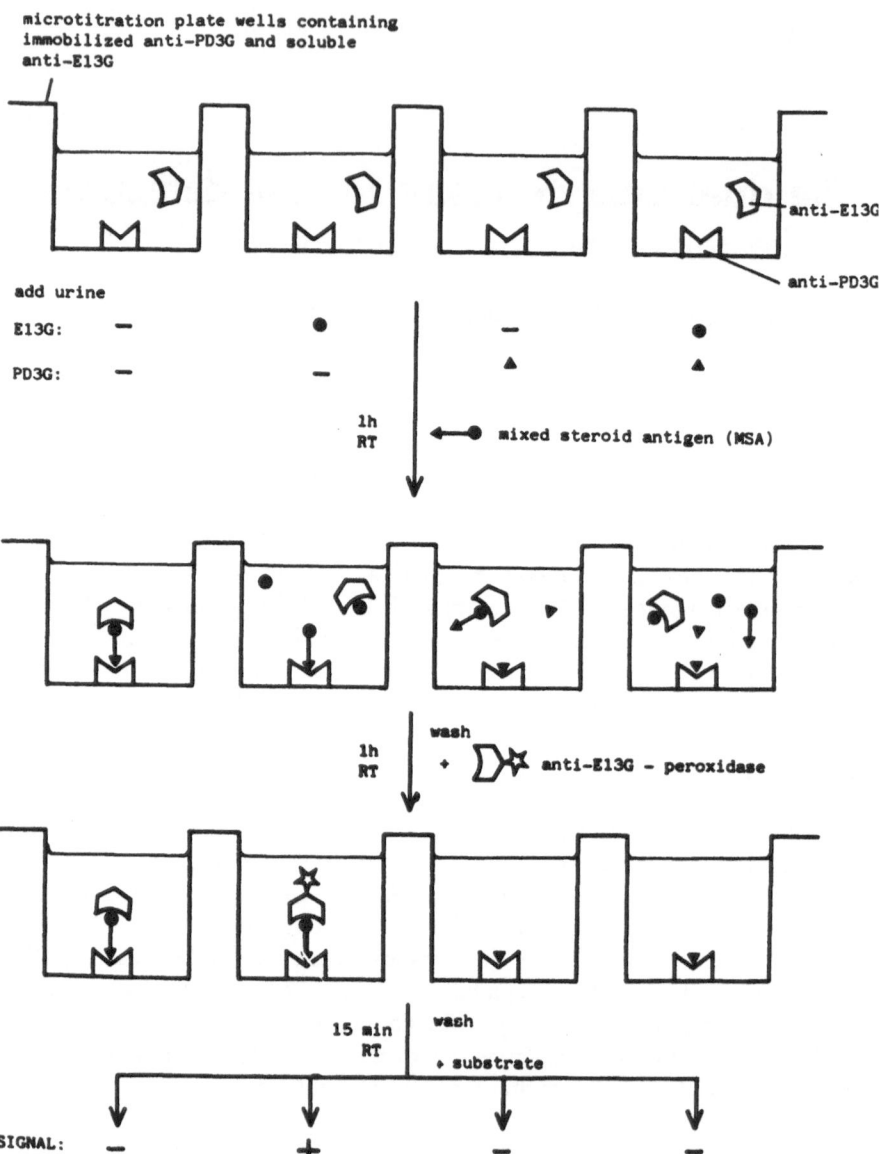

Figure 1 Dual Analyte Assay Protocol. (E₁-3-G, oestrone-3-glucuronide; PD-3-G, pregnanediol-3-glucuronide)

ratio in menstrual cycle urine samples. This is achieved by a three-stage reaction. The choice of the two substances as the preferred metabolites of E_2 and progesterone respectively was made on evidence generated within the WHO reproduction programme[1].

In the first stage, immobilized (anti-PD-3-G) antibody and soluble (anti-E_1-3-G) antibody can react with a di-steroid molecule, containing both E_1-3-G and PD-3-G functional groups, to give an immuno-complex 'sandwich' on a solid phase support. However, E_1-3-G in the sample can compete with one of these antigen–antibody reactions and PD-3-G therein can compete in the other.

The mechanism is best illustrated by describing responses in four extreme combinations, i.e. high or low concentrations of E_1-3-G and PD-3-G (Figure 1). Only one of these situations (high E_1-3-G, low PD-3-G) corresponds to the fertile period of the menstrual cycle. Under these conditions, the sandwich is only partially formed, leaving E_1-3-G functional groups protruding from the solid phase. This is not the case for the other three situations. The protruding groups are detected in the second and third stages, which involves reaction with enzyme labelled anti-E_1-3-G and substrate respectively. Thus, with a suitable substrate, a colour response is generated only when E_1-3-G is high and PD-3-G is low.

In its present form, the assay is performed in microtest plates, the plastic surfaces of the wells acting as solid phase support. The three stages can be completed within 2.5 hours and the colour end-point can be observed visually, although use of a plate reader is advisable. The technique is highly suitable for obtaining entire menstrual cycle profiles, since large numbers of samples can be handled with minimal technician time.

The Dual Analyte assay was investigated as part of WHO multi-centre trial of methods for the determination of the fertile period. Coded urine samples, representing some 17 menstrual cycles were analysed by this method. The data were examined to determine whether a suitable yes/no threshold, common to all cycles could be identified as a means of demarcating the fertile period.

MATERIALS AND METHODS

Menstrual cycle urines

Menstrual cycle urines were obtained from the WHO (Project No. 81909) courtesy of Prof. W. P. Collins, Kings College Hospital, Denmark Hill, London. The urines were early morning specimens obtained from 17 women and collected over a complete menstrual cycle. Quality control samples were also included, and all samples were stored at $-18\,°C$ prior to assay. Urine lutropin (LH) data, time of follicle rupture data (as determined by ultrasonography on 13 cycles) and sample codes were also supplied by the WHO following completion of the trial.

Reagents and assay protocol

Full details of reagents and methods have been described elsewhere[2].

Analysis of urine samples

A total of 538 coded urine samples were measured by the DAA method over 27 consecutive assays. An additional aliquot of a quality control urine sample collected at late follicular phase was also included in each assay. In one experiment to test the tolerance of the assay to sample dilution, standard mixtures of E_1-3-G and PD-3-G (corresponding to typical menstrual cycle concentrations) were assayed at 5, 10, 25 and 33.3-fold final dilution factors.

RESULTS

Between assay variation

The coded WHO samples contained multiple aliquots from four urine pools. Variation in results within each pool together with variation of the additional quality control urine are shown as follows:

Sample	No. of assays	Relative absorbance	CV%
Pool 1	21	59.5 ± 4.5	7.6
Pool 2	24	20.9 ± 2.6	12.6
Pool 3	25	29.6 ± 2.8	9.5
Male urine	4	37.6 ± 3.2	8.5
Late follicular phase	27	21.3 ± 2.6	12.1

Variation due to sample dilution factor

The potential advantage of measuring a ratio is that the signal should be independent of sample volume or dilution. For four different E_1-3-G/PD-3-G molar ratios, typical of menstrual cycle urine, the following mean relative absorbance values were obtained when measured at four different dilutions of sample:

Ratio	Relative absorbance	CV%
0.02	22.2 ± 2.2	9.9
0.04	28.5 ± 1.1	3.9
0.12	36.2 ± 3.4	9.4
0.20	43.9 ± 6.0	13.7

A remarkably consistent signal at each ratio was observed, despite there being a 6.66-fold dilution difference between the highest and lowest sample measured.

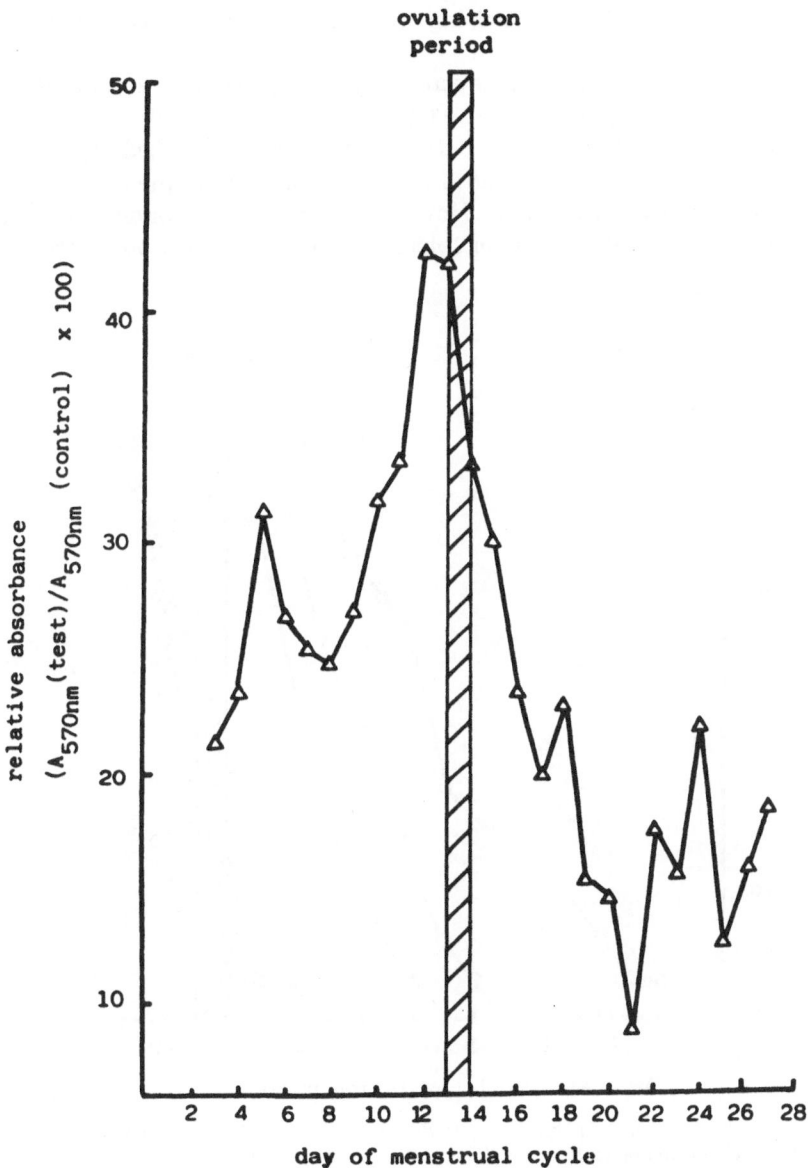

Figure 2 Dual Analyte analysis of a typical menstrual cycle

49

Menstrual cycle urines

The reference point in 13 cycles was designated day 0 by ultrasonography. One cycle was excluded from the study since no follicle was observed by ultra-sonography. Day 0 in the remaining cycles was designated according to urine LH data.

The relative absorbance profile across a typical cycle (Figure 2) showed a well defined surge over days -4 to -1 to reach a peak on day -1. This was followed by a rapid fall on day $+1$ onwards, to give a marked depression in absorbance values during the luteal phase. Minor peaks in the early follicular phase were observed in all cycles. However, the major peak dominated the cycle and provided a clear marker for follicular maturation. This observation was

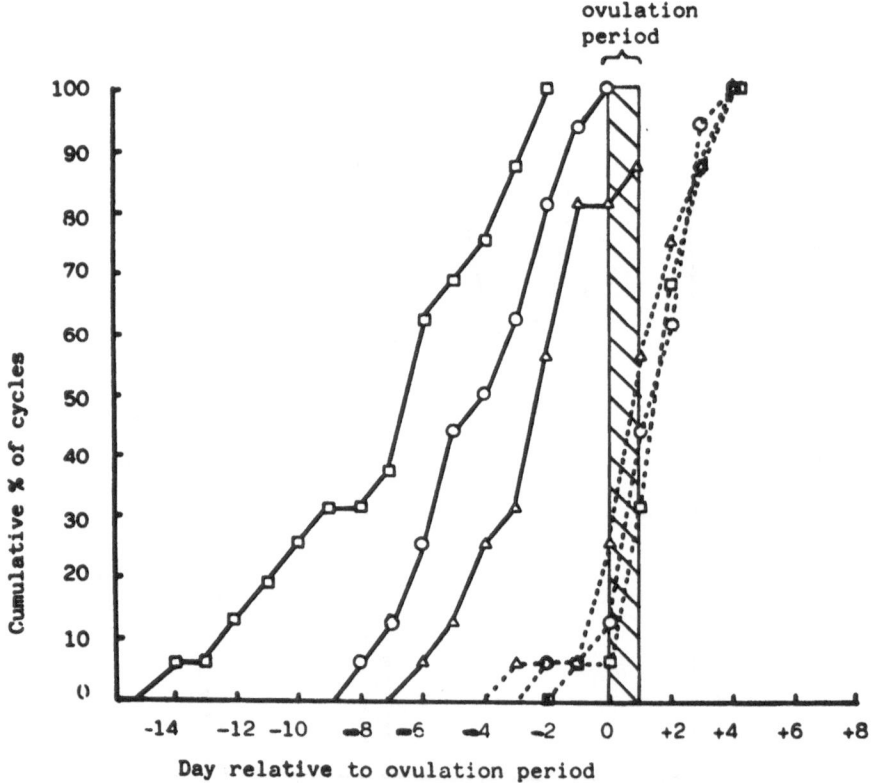

Figure 3 Ability of Dual Analyte Assay to demarcate the period of maximum fertility using a threshold value common to 16 cycles. (Cumulative % of cycles showing day of first increase in signal above threshold value (———) and first day of sustained depression in signal below threshold value (------). Data at 3 different threshold values are shown: □ 32%, ○ 35% and △ 40% A_{570nm} (test)/A_{570nm} (control) ($\times$ 100)

repeated for all cycles. Cumulative frequency curves were plotted in order to define a common threshold which (a) gave best warning of the start of the fertile period, (b) gave best estimate of predicting the time of ovulation and (c) gave best index of the end of the fertile period.

Cumulative percentage of cycles achieving a given index against day of cycle is shown in Figure 3. The indices being either the first day of a cycle when a given threshold was exceeded, or the first day in the cycle when a sustained depression in the relative absorbance was observed. Three threshold values are shown: 32%, 35% and 40% relative absorbance. Values above the threshold are referred to as positive and values below as negative.

Using the 35% threshold all cycles first gave a positive value between days −8 and 0. Better warning of ovulation was obtained by the lower threshold, with all cycles giving a positive value at or before day −2. However, at 32% threshold 30% of cycles gave 'false positive' values before day −8. By choosing a higher threshold (40%) there were no 'false positive' values before day −6 but in two cycles the threshold was not attained. On the other hand the 40% threshold produced the best estimate for predicting the time of ovulation; when 40% relative absorbance was first exceeded, ovulation occurred between 1 and 3 days later in 50% of cycles.

All three thresholds produced steep, very similar cumulative frequency curves for a decrease in signal; thus illustrating the dramatic fall in relative absorbance values following the ovulation period. From day +4 until the end of the cycle all subjects showed relative absorbance values below the 32% threshold. For the 16 subjects at the 35% threshold, the span of the 'fertile period' was 5.5 ± 2.6 days (range 1–9 days) corresponding to $19.7 \pm 8.7\%$ of the cycle length. At the 32% threshold the 'fertile period' was 7.3 ± 3.6 days (range 2–16 days) corresponding to $26.0 \pm 11.5\%$ of the cycle length.

DISCUSSION

Earlier reports have shown the value of measuring the E_1-3-G/PD-3-G ratio in menstrual cycle urine[1,3,4]. All these methods have required two separate measurements of the two analytes, and then computation of a ratio. More recently a method for the simultaneous measurement of E_1-3-G and PD-3-G has been described[5], but it involves two different end-points and interpolation of discrete concentrations before calculating a ratio.

The present method involves a single colour end-point, which is simultaneously responsive to both E_1-3-G and PD-3-G concentrations. No interpolations or computation of ratio values are required. The DAA also appears to be somewhat tolerant of sample dilution variation. An important finding in this study has been that it is possible to set an absorbance threshold which is common to all cycles, so that positive or negative changes about the threshold act as markers for the start or end of the fertile period. By raising or lowering this threshold value it is possible to tailor the DAA to particular applications.

For instance, as a method to assist in the management of infertility patients it may be useful to set a higher threshold (e.g. 40% relative absorbance). At the expense of missing a small proportion of cycles altogether, there is greater accuracy in predicting ovulation say, 1–3 days in advance.

As the basis of a home-use type kit for avoiding conception, a lower threshold would be preferable, (e.g. 32%). The method would then detect a rise in all cycles say, 2 or more days before ovulation, but at the expense of false positive results 8 days or more before ovulation. At either threshold the method is remarkably free from false positive values during most of the luteal phase.

The Dual Analyte assay has been shown to be a simple, reliable means of monitoring follicular function in women. With its visual, yes/no end-point, common to all cycles, it promises to be one of the best methods for determining the fertile period in women.

ACKNOWLEDGEMENTS

This work was made possible by Professor A. E. Kellie who devoted a large part of his scientific career to the study of steroid metabolism. The authors wish to thank Dr P. Samarajeewa of the Courtauld Institute of Biochemistry for the supply of steroid antisera. This investigation received financial support from the World Health Organization (Project No. 81094).

References

1. Adlercreutz, H., Brown, J., Collins, W., Goebelsman, U., Kellie, A., Campbell, H., Spieler, J. and Braissand, G. (1982). The measurement of urinary steroid glucuronides as indices of the fertile period in women. *J. Steroid Biochem.*, **17**, 695
2. Baker, T. S. and Coulson, W. F. (1983). Dual Analyte Assay. *Eur. Pat. Applic.* 83300569.7
3. Baker, T. S., Jennison, K. M. and Kellie, A. E. (1979). The direct radioimmunoassay of oestrogen glucuronides in human female urine. *Biochem. J.*, **177**, 729
4. Prendiville, W. and Baker, T. S. (1983). The relationship between the E/P index and the fertile period in women. Presented at the *XI World Congress on Fertility and Sterility*, June 26th–July 1st, Dublin
5. Weerasekera, D. A., Kim, J. B., Barnard, G. J. and Collins, W. P. (1983). Multiple immunoassay; the simultaneous measurement of two urinary steroid glucuronides as an index of ovarian function. *J. Steroid Biochem.*, **18**, 465

8
The relationship between the ratio of E_1-3-G/Pd-3-G and the fertile period

W. PRENDIVILLE AND T. S. BAKER

INTRODUCTION

Current methods of monitoring ovulation and the fertile period are imperfect. There is as yet no simple precise marker of ovulation. Modern methods of natural family planning aim to prevent conception by marking the fertile period surrounding ovulation. They are hampered by their subjective and/or retrospective nature. If a simple, reliable and objective marker of both the beginning and the end of the fertile period could be developed, these deficiencies might be overcome. We have investigated the relationship between the E/P index (oestrone-3-glucuronide/pregnanediol-3-glucuronide) and a defined 5 day period surrounding ovulation.

MATERIALS AND METHODS

In 43 ovulatory cycles, random daily urine samples were assayed for oestrone-3-glucuronide and pregnanediol-3-glucuronide using a solid phase radio-immuno-assay. Luteinizing hormone (LH) and creatinine (CR) values were measured from the same urine samples for 8 or more days surrounding ovulation. The onset of the LH/CR surge was taken to bear the most constant temporal relationship with ovulation[1], and was used as the marker of impending ovulation with which to compare the E/P index.

RESULTS

In 86% of cycles the E/P index values peaked before the onset of the LH/CR surge. Various features of the E/P index pattern were studied and, in particular, aspects of the pre-ovulatory rise which occurred in every cycle.

The threshold value of 30 (T 30) predated the onset of the LH/CR surge in every cycle studied. This signal did not first occur at a constant time relative to LH but appeared at various times during the early follicular phase. Also in some cycles the E/P index values dropped below the signal T 30 before the end of the 5 day peri-ovulatory period. In order to accommodate these deficiencies and recognise the entire fertile period in every cycle it is necessary to modify interpretation of the T 30 signal. That is to say were a woman/couple to recognise a potentially fertile period whenever the signal T 30 was reached and to maintain sexual continence until 3 days after the E/P index had fallen below the T 30 signal, then the fertile period would be recognised in all of the 43 cycles studied. However, this would mean sexual abstinence for a mean of 48% of any cycle (range: 19%–86%).

DISCUSSION

The E/P index has considerable potential advantages over other methods of monitoring ovarian function and the menstrual cycle that are currently in use. First of all, much of the scope for subjective error that exists with basal body temperature and mucus evaluation is removed. Secondly, the expense and inconvenience of endometrial biopsy or venepuncture is avoided. Urine is easily and conveniently collected. The E/P index is a modified ratio. The use of a ratio principle has practical advantages. It negates the need for volume or concentration markers such as 24 hour collections or creatinine estimations. The use of the particular ratio of oestrone-3-glucuronide/pregnanediol-3-glucuronide has a further advantage. With this ratio the values found in the early and late follicular phases are distinguishable from those found in the luteal phase. This is because in the follicular phases (early and late) the rising E/P index is actually a reflection of oestrone-3-glucuronide with pregnanediol acting as a concentration marker. Whereas in the luteal phase the values of pregnanediol are significantly elevated thereby depressing the E/P index, within the peri-ovulatory period the E/P index peaks.

The E/P index is expected to have an application in two general areas: the subfertility clinic and as part of a method of natural family planning. It is recognised that the true effectiveness and acceptability of such a method will only be determined by a properly constructed clinical trial.

References

1. WHO Task Force on Methods for the Determination of the Fertile Period, Special Programme of Research, Development and Research Training in Human Reproduction. (1980). Temporal relationships between ovulation and defined changes in the concentration of plasma estradiol – 17β, luteinizing hormone, follicle-stimulating hormone, and progesterone. 1. Probit analysis. *Am. J. Obstet. Gynecol.*, **138**, 383

9
Prolactin, gonadotrophins and oestrogen levels in lactating puerperae and in non-lactating puerperae treated with metergoline or bromocriptine

R. DI MICCO, A. SARTANI, A. CUCCI, A. E. PONTIROLI
AND E. ZANARDI

INTRODUCTION

The post-partum period in lactating women is characterized by hyperprolactinaemia and infertility. Investigations aimed at elucidating the factors causing the temporary anovulatory state yielded different results.

It has been claimed that prolactin acted at the ovarian level[1] or induced pituitary refractoriness[2]. Others suggested that lactation itself was the causal factor[3]. A multifactorial mechanism has also been postulated[4].

Bromocriptine[3] and metergoline[5] are effective in suppressing puerperal lactation but might act through different mechanisms. We, therefore, investigated the effect of these two drugs on the prolactin and the gonadotropins during the early post-partum period, in comparison to lactating women.

SUBJECTS AND METHODS

Twenty-eight parturient women after a full-term pregnancy were evaluated: 13 women (mean age of 28.9 ± 1.4 years) breast-fed, and 15 women (mean age of 30.0 ± 1.3) did not for either medical or personal reasons. They were randomly allocated to either metergoline 12 mg/d ($n = 9$) or bromocriptine 5 mg/d ($n = 6$) treatment for 14 days each. Prolactin, FSH, LH, β-HCG and oestradiol levels were determined on days 1, 3, 7 and 14 after delivery. LHRH test with 100 μg i.v. was performed at the same time on days 1, 7 and 14.

The test started immediately after either termination of breast-feeding or medication. Progesterone levels were determined prior to the second postpartum menses.

Statistical analysis was performed on basal levels of each hormone and on the FSH and LH secretory areas (ΔAUC, mIU/ml/120 min, calculated by the trapezoidal method), by the two-tailed Student's 't' test for paired or unpaired data.

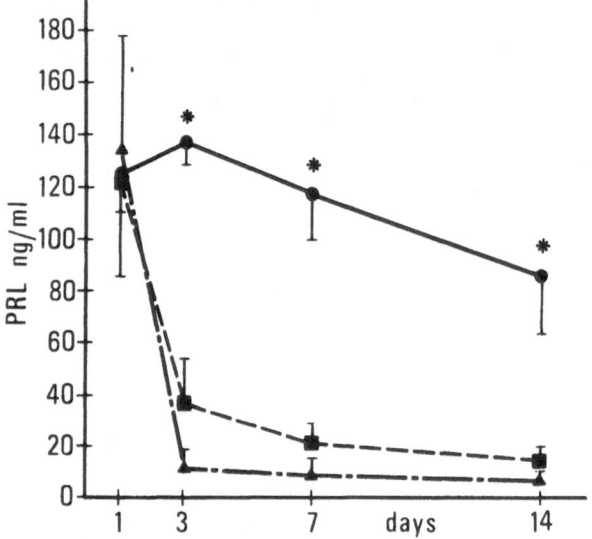

Figure 1   Serum prolactin (PRL, ng/ml) levels observed 1, 3, 7 and 14 days after delivery in breast feeding puerperae (l, ●—●) and in puerperae treated with metergoline (m, ■--■) and with bromocriptine (b, ▲-.-▲). Means ± SEM* p < 0.05 vs. puerperae treated with the two drugs

Table 1   Patient protocol

	Duration of lactation (days)	Time from delivery to 1st menses (days)	No. of patients with ovulatory progesterone levels (2nd cycle)
1. Lactation	56.3 ± 13.1 (15–153)	89.6 ± 13.1 (32–182)	1/13
2. Metergoline		57.3 ± 5.4 (38–65)	5/8*
3. Bromocriptine		58.5 ± 7.1 (42–69)	1/6

*Significant vs. lactating women (χ^2 test), not significant vs. bromocriptine
Mean ± SEM, range in parenthesis

RESULTS

The first menstrual period in lactating women occurred 89.6 ± 13.1 days (mean ± SEM) after delivery in comparison to 57.3 ± 5.4 and 58.5 ± 7.1 in the metergoline and bromocriptine groups respectively. Ovulatory progesterone

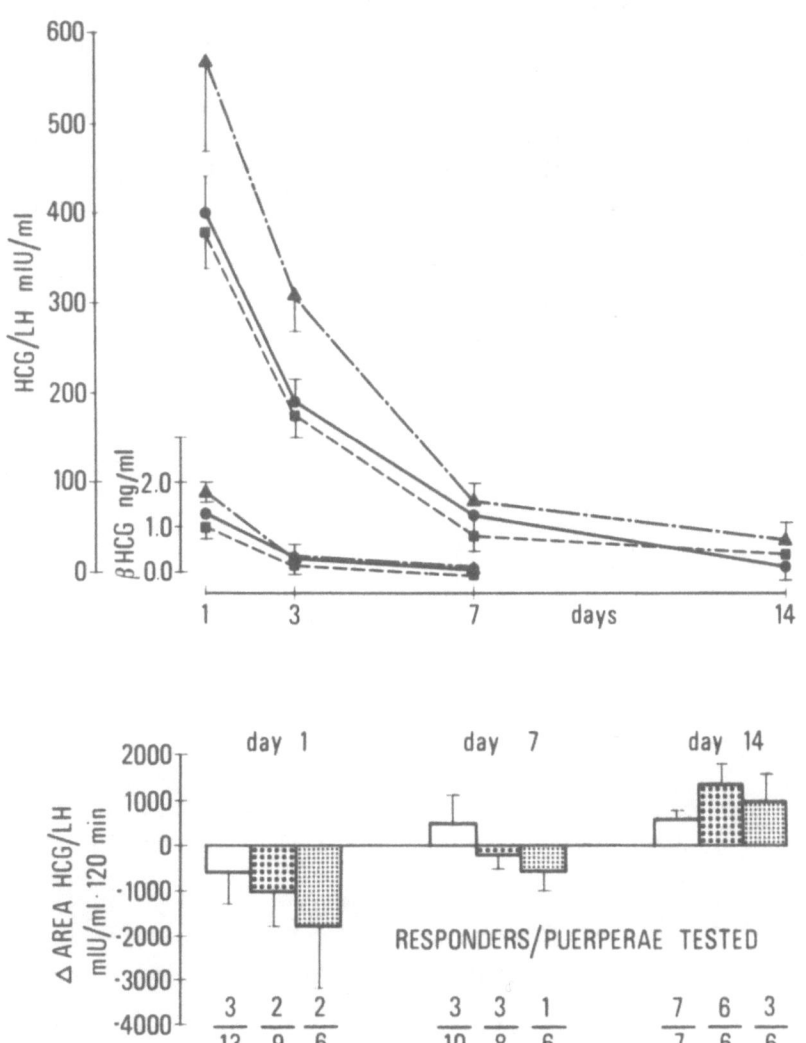

Figure 2 (a) Serum hCG/LH (mIU/ml) and βhCG (ng/ml) levels and hCG/LH response to LHRH (Δ area hCG/LH, mIU/ml/120 min) observed 1, 3, 7 and 14 days after delivery in breast-feeding puerperae (l, ●——●; □) and (b) in puerperae treated with metergoline (m, ■ -- ■ ; □) and with bromocriptine (b, ▲ -.- ▲ ; ◇). Means ± SEM

levels were found during the second post-partum cycle in 1 out of 13 lactating women, 5 out of 8 ($p<0.05$ vs. lactating women) and 1 out of 6 in the metergoline and bromocriptine groups respectively (Table 1).

Prolactin secretion and lactation were equally suppressed by the two drugs (Figure 1). LH/β-hCG levels diminished in all three groups (Figure 2) in a similar way and the response to LHRH was evident on day 14. The percentage of responders was higher in the lactating and metergoline treated women than in the bromocriptine group. FSH basal levels (Figure 3) followed a different pattern in non-lactating treated puerperae as compared to lactating women. Plasma levels did not tend to diminish in the treated women and were higher than in the lactating females (significantly for bromocriptine vs. lactating). On the other hand, FSH response to LHRH was similar in all three groups and appeared earlier than the LH response.

Oestradiol levels (Figure 4) probably followed FSH secretion. In fact, there was a decrease in all groups until day 7, with a significant increase in serum levels from day 7 to day 14 only in the non-lactating women.

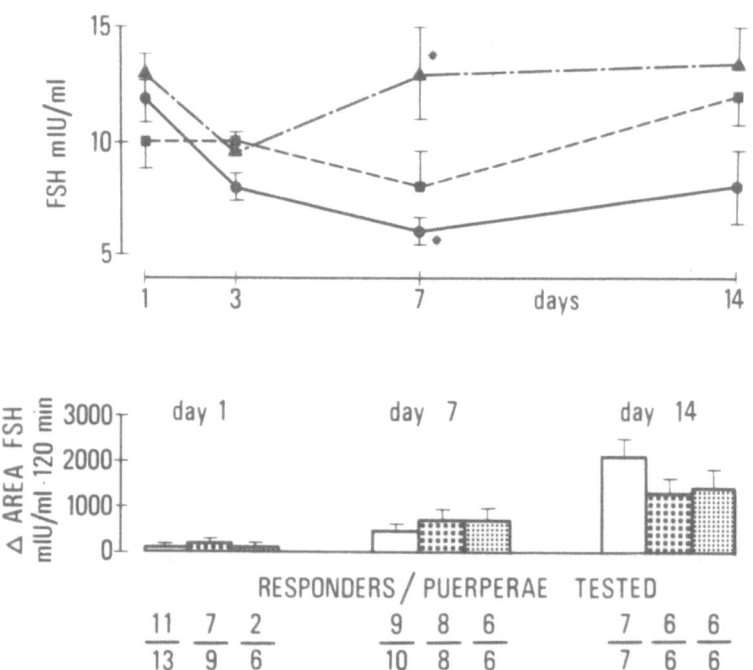

Figure 3 (a) Serum FSH (mIU/ml) levels and FSH response to LHRH (Δ area FSH, mIU/ml/ 120 min) observed 1, 3, 7 and 14 days after delivery in breast-feeding puerperae (l, ●——●, □) and (b) in puerperae treated with metergoline (m, ■ -- ■) and with bromocriptine (b, ▲ --- ▲ ; □). Means ± SEM

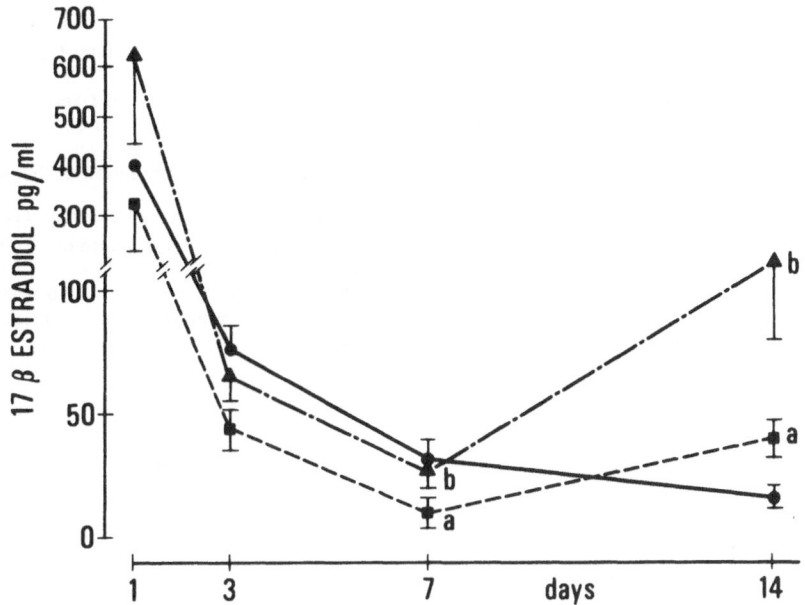

Figure 4 Serum 17-β oestradiol (pg/ml) levels observed 1, 3, 7 and 14 days after delivery in breast-feeding puerperae (l, ●—● ;) and in puerperae treated with metergoline (m, ■ -- ■ ;) and with bromocriptine (b, ▲ -.- ▲ ;). Means ± SEM metergoline day 14 vs day 7, $p < 0.01$; bromocriptine day 14 vs day 7, $p < 0.001$

CONCLUSIONS

1. Both drugs were equally effective in lowering prolactin and suppressing lactation. Menstruation returned earlier in the non-lactating women. The possible earlier return of ovulation in the metergoline group requires further investigation.

2. FSH basal levels seem to behave differently in non-lactating treated women in comparison to lactating women, and that might cause the early rise in E_2 levels. FSH response to pharmacological dose of LHRH is seen quite early, before that of LH, and does not seem to depend either on PRL levels or on the drug used.

3. LH basal levels were similar in all groups. The response to LHRH was similar in all groups in its pattern and amount, although the percentage of responders was somewhat lower in the bromocriptine group.

4. We may speculate that ovarian refractoriness due to high PRL levels is one of the factors responsible for the anovulatory state.

References

1. Bonnar, J., Franklin, M., Nott, P. N. and McNeilly, A. S. (1975). Effect of breast-feeding on pituitary–ovarian function after childbirth. *Br. Med. J.*, **4**, 82
2. Keye, W. R. and Jaffe, R. B. (1976). Changing patterns of FSH and LH response to gonadotropin-releasing hormone in the puerperium. *J. Clin. Endocrinol. Metab.*, **42**, 1133
3. Del Pozo, E., Varga, L., Schulz, K. D., Künzig, H. J., Marbach, P., Lopez del Campo, G. and Eppenberger, U. (1975). Pituitary and ovarian response patterns to stimulation in the post-partum and in galactorrhea–amenorrhea. *Obstet. Gynecol.*, **46**, 539
4. Tyson, J. E., Freedman, R. S., Perez, A., Zacur, H. A. and Zanartu, J. (1976). Significance of the secretion of human prolactin and gonadotropin for puerperal lactational infertility. *CIBA Foundation Symposium 45, Excerpta Medica, Amsterdam*, 49
5. Falsetti, L., Voltolini, A. M., Pollini, C. and Pontiroli, A. E. (1982). A study of prolactin, follicle-stimulating hormone, and luteinizing hormone in puerperium: spontaneous variations and the effect of metergoline. *Fertil. Steril.*, **37**, 397

10
PGE$_2$ versus methyl-ergometrin in the puerperium. Influence in uterine involution and on lactation patterns

W. GRÜNBERGER AND G. GERSTNER

INTRODUCTION

Recently a 'renaissance in breast feeding' has been noted in industrialized western countries[1-4]. Human milk is now generally regarded to be superior to artificial milks.

Methylergometrin, which is widely used in the puerperium has been shown to have a negative influence on lactation[5-7]. Recent studies have failed to confirm that methylergometrin accelerates the involution of the uterus, increases the secretion of the lochiae and consequently results in a decreased infectious morbidity[8, 9]. Therefore, some authors have suggested stopping the routine administration of methylergometrin in the puerperium, and of using uterotonics without negative side effects on lactation and then only when indicated. The aim of this study was to compare methylergometrin and PGE$_2$.

MATERIAL AND METHODS

Eighty puerperal women were included in a prospective randomized clinical trial. From the first to the fifth postpartum day either 0.5 mg PGE$_2$ (Prostin-E$_2$ tablets) or 0.125 mg methylergometrin (Methergin) were administered three times a day. Both groups were comparable with regard to age, parity and mode of delivery. All patients delivered spontaneously at term. Excluded were pregnancies with risk, multiple pregnancies, breech deliveries and cases in which labour was induced by oxytocin.

We examined the number and intensity of pain of the uterine contractions, height of the uterine fundus in the puerperium, lochial secretion, frequency of the stools, heart rate, blood pressure, body temperature and the onset of lactation and the amount of milk. The uterine involution and the lochial secretion were estimated according to a given score.

Therapeutic failures in each group were allocated to the other treatment-group on the morning of the fourth day. Quantitative data were analysed with the Student t-test, qualitative data with the χ^2-test and individual comparisons with the Dixon-Mood test.

RESULTS

On the fourth postpartum day the uterine involution was insufficient in nine patients from the PGE_2 group and in 10 patients from the methylergometrin group. In the latter group three patients had a temperature over 37.5 °C as compared to only one patient in the PGE_2 group. According to a 'cross-over' trial a total of 19 therapeutic failures was switched over to the other treatment group.

The other regime was only successful in one of nine cases when the treatment was switched to methylergometrin, in comparison to 8 of 10 cases when the treatment was switched to PGE_2 after failure of methylergometrin. This difference is statistically significant ($p < 0.01$).

Patients treated with one drug from the first to the fifth postpartum day ('non-cross-over-sample') showed the following results:

(1) A statistically significant difference was found only for pain on the third day postpartum. Patients in the methylergometrin group experienced more pain on that day. A tendency to more frequent and painful contractions was also recorded on the fourth day in this group.

(2) The uterine fundus, which in the PGE_2 group was higher on the first postpartum day, was distinctly lower than in the methylergometrin group on day 5.

(3) On the second and third postpartum day a tendency towards an increased lochial secretion was noted in the PGE_2 group. Stools were more frequent on day 4 and 5 in the PGE_2 group.

(4) The milk-volume was significantly higher in patients in the PGE_2 group from the third postpartum day onwards. In the PGE_2 group the total milk-volume from the first to the fifth postpartum day exceeded the methylergometrin group by 345 ml or 75% ($p < 0.01$) (Table 1). No differences were found concerning the heart rate, the systolic and diastolic blood pressure and the mean body temperature.

Table 1 Results of the 'non-crossover-sample' onset of lactation, amount of milk

Onset of lactation (day)	PGE_2 (ml)	Methylergometrin (ml)	Significance n.s.
1	1.3 ± 5.0		n.s.
2	24.5 ± 48.5	19.2 ± 47.5	n.s.
3	127.1 ± 116.1	54.3 ± 78.9	$p < 0.01$
4	313.2 ± 193.2	168.3 ± 162.9	$p < 0.01$
5	370.6 ± 186.1	248.1 ± 190.4	$p < 0.05$
1–5	836.7 ± 487	490.8 ± 398	$p < 0.01$

mean ± SD

DISCUSSION

Like all ergot-alkaloids methylergometrin has a dopaminergic effect. Low doses of 0.25–0.5 mg orally cause a decrease in prolactin levels up to 44% which persist for 4 hours. This decrease in serum-prolactin levels is considered by most authors as the cause of diminished lactation seen in methylergometrin treatment[5-7]. This question, however, is not entirely clear as the required plasma prolactin concentration for sufficient lactation[10] is only 30 ng/ml.

From the results of our study we cannot conclude whether methylergometrin influences the milk-volume negatively, or if the increased lactation was stimulated by the administration of PGE_2 due to its oxytocic effect. However, in our prospective randomized study nearly all the examined parameters were found to be in favour of PGE_2.

References

1. Gerstner, G. and Grünberger, W. (1980). Faktoren, die das Bruststillen beeinflussen können. Z. Geburtsh. Perinat., 184, 70–75
2. Gerstner, G., Grünberger, W. and Leodolter, S. (1982). Ursachen der Laktationshemmung im Frühwochenbett. Z. Geburtsch. Perinat., 186, 97–100
3. Müller, H. G. (1979). Die Vorteile des Stillens und die Stillprobleme in der Neugeborenenperiode. Med. Diss. Heidelberg
4. Winikoff, B. and Baer, E. C. (1980). The obstetricians' opportunity: translating 'breast is best' from theory to practice. Am. J. Obstet. Gynecol., 138, 105–7
5. Canales, E. S., Garrido, J. I., Zarate, A., Mason, M. and Soria, J. (1976). Effect of ergonovine on prolactin secretion and milk let-down. Obstet. Gynecol., N.Y., 48, 228–9
6. Martius, J., Loock, W. and Brandau, H. (1981). Wirkung einer Methylergometringabe im Wochenbett auf Prolaktingehalt und Stilleistung. Gynäk. Rdsch., 21, 118–20
7. Varga, L., Lutterbeck, P. M. and Pryor, S. S. (1972). Suppression of puerperal lactation with an ergot alkaloid: a double-blind study. Br. Med. J., 3, 743–4
8. Arabin, B., Rüttgers, H., Leucht, W. and Kubli, F. (1981). Bedeutung der routinemäßigen uterotonischen Behandlung im Wochenbett. Gynäk. Rdsch., 21, 116–17
9. Dörner, G., Faber, G., Tabatt, K. and Wurzbach, A. (1979). Laktationhemmung durch frühpostpartale Gaben von Methylergobrevin. Zentbl. Gynäk., 101, 25–8
10. Del Pozo, E., Del Re, R. B. and Hinselmann, M. (1975). Lack of effect of methyl-ergonovine on postpartum lactation. Am. J. Obstet. Gynecol., 121, 845–6

Section 2

Steroid Contraception

11
Comparative randomized double-blind study of high dosage ethinyloestradiol vs. ethinyloestradiol-norgestrel combination in postcoital hormonal contraception

M. R. VAN SANTEN AND A. A. HASPELS

ABSTRACT

Over the last 15 years high dosages of ethinyloestradiol (5 mg EE_2) for 5 consecutive days have been used to prevent pregnancy after a single unprotected intercourse. Recently the use of a combination of 200 μg ethinyloestradiol and 2 mg dl-norgestrel (EE_2 + norg) divided into two equal parts given within a 12 hour period has been proposed as an effective alternative.

Efficacy and tolerance were compared by the random administration of sets of plain capsules containing either treatment, or placebo taken for 5 days, with two capsules the first day.

Efficacy: in 466 cases, with a follow-up of 94.5% 2 pregnancies occurred in the 5 mg EE_2 group ($n = 226$), and one pregnancy was observed in the EE_2 + norg group ($n = 240$); this gave an overall corrected pregnancy rate of, respectively, 0.9% and 0.4%. Analysis of efficacy, by calculating the expected number of pregnancies by day of coitus, revealed an expected number of pregnancies in the 5 mg EE_2 group of 11.9 versus the observed 2 pregnancies. The pregnancy rates respectively were 6.5% and 1.1%, showing a statistically significant difference (χ^2 test $p < 0.001$). Similarly for the EE_2 + norg group the number of expected pregnancies was 11, while only 1 was observed. The pregnancy rates were respectively 5.5% and 0.5%, also a statistically significant difference ($p < 0.001$).

Side effects: nausea-only was noted by 59.1% in the 5 mg EE_2 group ($n = 149$), while 54.0% was observed with the EE_2 + norg ($n = 170$) method. Nausea and vomiting was seen respectively in 20.8% and 15.8%. These figures do not differ significantly (student's *t*-test).

These data confirm the efficacy of both methods in preventing conception after a single unprotected sexual encounter. Since the recently proposed alternative morning-after medication (which is only taken on one day) this is the preferred method.

INTRODUCTION

In the United States, Canada and Great Britain the use of a new alternative hormonal postcoital treatment is becoming generally accepted, the so called Yuzpe's method. This regimen employing 200 μg ethinyloestradiol and 2 mg dl-norgestrel within 72 hours after a single unprotected sexual encounter has been shown to be effective in several studies[1-3]. Some sceptism has been expressed in a British study however, where some failures were observed after midcycle unprotected exposure using this new method[4]. In a larger study of 692 women a reduction of expected pregnancies by 84% was observed, but a call was made for a randomized double-blind study to further compare the efficacy of this new method using the high dosage oestrogen (5 mg ethinyloestradiol for 5 days) regimen currently used in most countries in Europe[5]. A half-way evaluation of such a study was published earlier[6].

MATERIALS AND METHODS

In 466 women requesting postcoital hormonal contraception after one single unprotected sexual encounter, treatment with high dosage ethinyloestradiol (5 mg EE_2) or 200 μg ethinyloestradiol and 2 mg dl-norgestrel (EE_2 + norg) was randomly given. Six plain capsules were wrapped into a strip, and the patients instructed to take the first two capsules within the first 24 hours, twelve hours apart, and one capsule daily for the next 4 days. The effective compound-containing capsules were added to similar looking placebo capsules so that the final appearance of each strip containing either regimen was identical.

Interval time after coitus

Since 5 mg EE_2 treatment has been shown to be most effective if started within 24 hours postcoitum[7], this recommendation also applies to the EE_2 + norg treated group for reason of comparison.

RESULTS

In total 466 women were included in this study, with a follow-up of 94.5%. With the 5 mg EE_2 regimen 226 women were treated, while 240 used the EE_2 + norg treatment.

Efficacy

Several problems arise if an attempt is made to properly demonstrate the efficacy. Factors such as lack of a placebo control group, the lack of proof of fertility of the male partner and the patient herself, and the frequent lack of knowledge about her own menstrual history hamper proper analysis.

Derived from three studies on the probability of conception on a given day of the menstrual cycle a weighted average ratio on the probability by day of coitus is available[8] and is represented in Table 1.

Table 1 Pregnancy ratio per menstrual cycle day

Day	−9	−8	−7	−6	−5	−4	−3	−2	−1
Ratio	0	.001	.007	.025	.055	.104	.146	.169	.173

Day Ovulation	0	+1	+2	+3	+4	+5	+6 and over	
Ratio	.141	.091	.049	.019	.005	.001	0	

With such a ratio the expected pregnancy rate for a group of women with a known menstrual cycle and day of coitus can be estimated. In order to make comparable calculations of the probability of conception, those menstrual cycle lengths not equal to 28 days had to be aligned. The menstrual cycle day-number

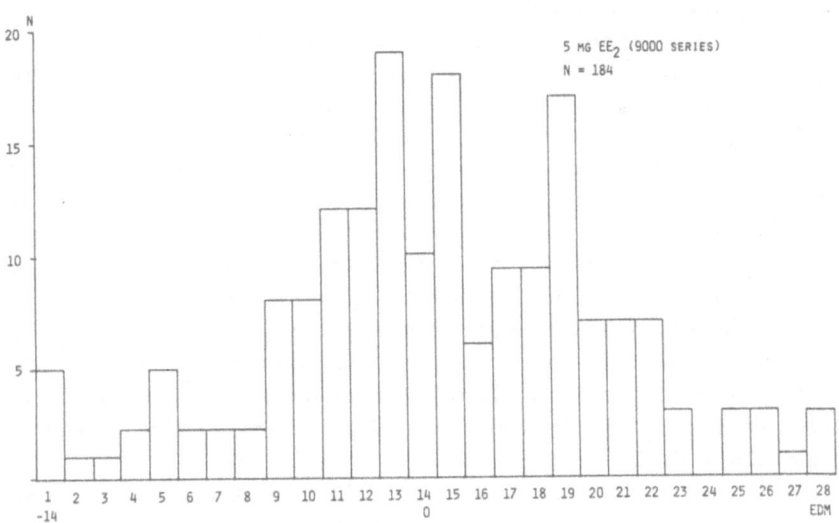

MENSTRUAL CYCLE DAY OF COITUS IN RELATION TO EXPECTED DAY OF MENSTRUATION

Figure 1

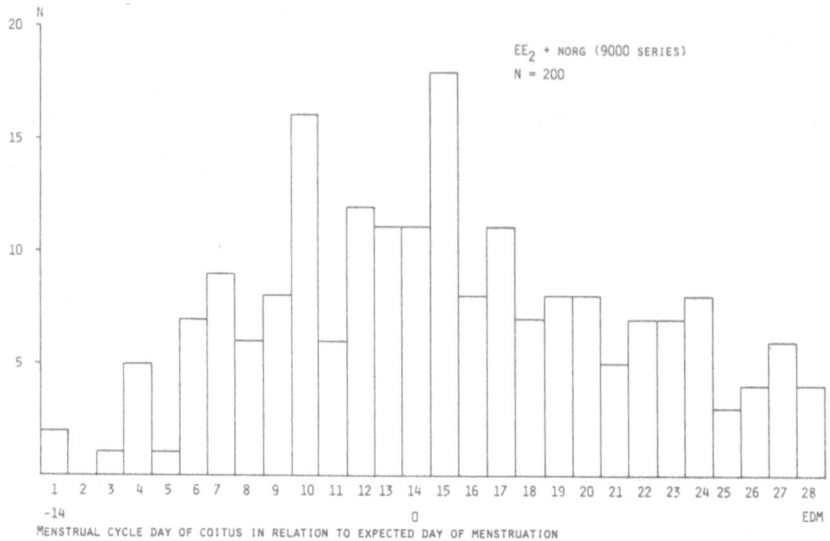

Figure 2

of the coitus was substracted from the woman's average menstrual cycle length. This 'coital luteal length' was then in turn substracted from a standard menstrual length of 28 days. This figure gives the 'recalculated menstrual cycle day of coitus' and is used for the calculation of the probability of pregnancy. For each day of the menstrual cycle the number of expected pregnancies was estimated.

Figures 1 and 2 show the distribution of the menstrual cycle day of coitus in the 5 mg EE_2 group ($n = 184$) and the EE_2 + norg group ($n = 200$), respectively.

In the 5 mg EE_2 group ($n = 226$), two pregnancies were observed. The overall pregnancy rate for all participating women was 0.9%. However, when only women with a regular menstrual cycle are collected, a comparative evaluation of expected and observed pregnancy rates can be made (Tables 2 and 3). In the 5 mg EE_2 group 184 patients were evaluated in such a way. We expected 11.9 pregnancies, however only two were observed. These pregnancy rates of 6.5% and 1.5% differ statistically significantly (χ^2-test $p < 0.001$).

In the EE_2 + norg group ($n = 240$), two pregnancies were observed. However, the second patient informed us on her questionnaire that she had several unprotected sexual encounters before she took the morning-after capsules; we, therefore, excluded her from further evaluation. The corrected overall pregnancy rate is 0.4%.

Comparative evaluation of expected and observed pregnancy rates in the EE_2 + norg group ($n = 200$), gave 11 pregnancies expected and 1 observed, revealing a statistically significant difference (χ^2-test $p < 0.001$) between, respectively, 5.5% and 0.5%.

Table 2 Observed vs expected pregnancies by day of coitus and in 5 mg EE₂ (‡ double-blind study vs EE₂+norg) group

	−13 to −8	−7	−6	−5	−4	−3	−2	−1	0	+1	+2	+3	+4	+5 to 14	Total	Rate*
							Day of coitus									
Expected	0	0	0.1	0.4	0.8	1.7	2	3.3	1.4	1.6	0.3	0.2	0.1	0	11.9	6.5
Observed	0	0	0	0	0	0	0	0	0	0	0	1	0	1	2	1.1
Total	0	2	2	8	8	12	12	19	10	18	6	10	10	51	184	

*per 100 women χ^2_{12} p<0.001
N=184

Table 3 Observed vs expected pregnancies by day of coitus and in EE₂+norg (‡ double-blind study vs 5 mg EE₂) group

	−13 to −8	−7	−6	−5	−4	−3	−2	−1	0	+1	+2	+3	+4	+5 to 14	Total	Rate*
							Day of coitus									
Expected	0	0.1	0.2	0.4	1.7	0.9	2.0	1.9	1.6	1.6	0.4	0.2	0	0	11	5.5
Observed	0	0	0	0	0	0	1	0	0	0	0	0	0	0	1	0.5
Total	17	9	6	8	16	6	12	11	11	18	8	11	7	60	200	

*per 100 women χ^2_{12} p<0.001
N=200

71

Side effects

Information on side effects in the 5 mg EE_2 group was obtained in 149 women. Nausea only was noted by 59.1% while nausea and vomiting occurred in 20.8%. In the EE_2 + norg group ($n = 170$) nausea was observed in 54.0%, and nausea plus vomiting in 15.8%. These figures do not differ significantly (student's *t*-test).

CONCLUSION

This study confirms the efficacy in preventing pregnancy by two different post-coital hormonal treatments given within 24 hours postcoitum. Since the Yuzpe's regimen requires only 24 hours of treatment, this new treatment is preferred for postcoital hormonal interception.

References

1. Yuzpe, A. A. (1979). Post Coital Contraception *Int. J. Gynaecol. Obstet.*, 16, 497–501
2. Rowlands, S. and Guillebaud, J. (1981). Postcoital contraception, a review. *Br. J. Fam. Plann.*, 7, 3–7
3. Rowlands, S. (1982). Morning-after pills. *Br. Med. J.*, 285, 322–3
4. Tully, B. (1983). Postcoital contraception, a study. *Br. J. Fam. Plann.*, 8, 119–24
5. Yuzpe, A. A., Smith, R. P. and Rademaker, A. W. (1982). A multicenter clinical investigation employing ethinylestradiol combined with dl-norgestrel as a postcoital contraceptive agent. *Fertil. Steril.*, 37, 508–13
6. Van Santen, M. R. and Haspels, A. A. (1982). Comparative randomized double-blind study of high dosage ethinylestradiol versus ethinylestradiol and norgestrel combination in postcoital contraception. *Acta Endocrinol.*, 99, 246
7. Haspels, A. A. (1976). Interception: postcoital estrogens in 3016 women. *Contraception*, 14, 375–81 and *Obstet. Gynecol. Surv.*, (1977). 32, 231–2
8. Dixon, G. W., Schlesselman, J. J., Ory, H. H. and Blye, R. P. (1980). Ethinylestradiol and conjugated estrogens as postcoital contraceptives. *J. Am. Med. Assoc.*, 244, 1336–40.

12
The contraceptive effect of the pill is not mediated by the quality of the peritoneal fluid

L. A. SCHELLEKENS, P. X. J. M. BOUCKAERT AND
M. F. H. A. VAN DER CRUYS

INTRODUCTION

Our interest in the peritoneal fluid was raised by the work of Maathuis in Edinburgh, in the early 1970s, later followed by the group of Koninckx in Louvain.

Contributions to the composition of the peritoneal fluid can be made by the secretory products of the uterus and tubes, exudations of the peritoneum, exudations through the surface of the ovaries, more importantly by the surface of the preovulatory follicle, and finally at ovulation by the follicular fluid.

In our institute Bouckaert studied different aspects of the peritoneal fluid in a large group of normal fertile women. A part of this study is presented by Bouckaert elsewhere in this congress[1].

The contraceptive effect of the pill is known to act at the ovarian level (causing anovulation), at the endometrial level, (causing atrophy), as well as at the cervical level, where the mucus blocks the penetration of spermatozoa.

In 1977 Koch and co-workers[2] demonstrated that the behaviour of spermatozoa in peritoneal fluid was of prognostic value in patients with infertility. This different behaviour of spermatozoa could be explained by the different biochemical qualities of the peritoneal fluid; perhaps by the presence or absence of macrophages. Therefore, we studied the behaviour of spermatozoa in the peritoneal fluid of women with proven fertility, one group acting as controls, with another group taking oral contraceptives. We investigated the question

73

whether the contraceptive effect of the pill could be enhanced by a blocking effect of the peritoneal fluid for spermatozoa.

MATERIAL AND METHODS

All samples of peritoneal fluid were taken during laparoscopy under direct visual control.

After storage at a temperature of 4°C, a spermatozoa-penetration-meter test (SPM) after Kremer was performed[3] within 5 days. The reservoir was filled with fresh human semen of normal fertile quality, the capillary in this experiment was peritoneal fluid. After 30 minutes and 2 hours the number of spermatozoa was counted at 100 times magnification at 3 and 5 cm in the capillary. The test results were scored described by Kremer, as modified by Roumen[4] (Table 1).

Table 1 SPM score following Roumen[4]

		Number of spermatozoa	Distance (cm)	Time (hours)
Good	5	⩾1	5	0.5
		>10	5	2
Sufficient	4	⩾1	5	2
Moderate	3	⩾1	<3	2
Bad	2	⩾1	<3	2
Negative	1	0	3	2

In the control group 116 subjects were tested, some before, and some after ovulation. The moment of ovulation was calculated by repeated assays of FSH, LH, oestradiol and progesterone.

We then tested the peritoneal fluid in 32 patients who came for laparoscopy while they were taking oral contraceptives. Only included in the study were those women who had taken their pill during the last 3 days before laparoscopy. All had a combination type of pill, no patients on sequential pills or step-up pills were accepted into the study.

RESULTS

The results of the SPM-tests in the control group and the oral contraceptive group are shown in Table 2.

In the control group all 116 subjects had some peritoneal fluid. In this group the SPM was scored as good in 50 subjects, as sufficient in 54, as moderate in 10 and as negative in 2.

In the oral contraceptive group of 32 patients, 12 of them had no peritoneal fluid; in 20 subjects, between 0.5 and 35 ml peritoneal fluid was recovered

Table 2 SPM test in peritoneal fluid

	Score	Control group (n = 116)	Oral contraceptive group (n = 20)
Good	5	50	17
Sufficient	4	54	3
Moderate	3	10	0
Bad	2	0	0
Negative	1	2	0

with a mean of 6.8 ml (SD 8.24, SEM 4.5). This quantity corresponds with the findings in our control group during the preovulatory phase of the menstrual cycle. In 17 of these 20 subjects, the SPM-score was good; the other 3 scored as sufficient.

CONCLUSION

From this study we conclude that women on the pill have a relatively small quantity of peritoneal fluid, corresponding to the volume of peritoneal fluid in the preovulatory phase of the cycle.

Sperm migration in the peritoneal fluid, measured by the SPM-test, was as good in the patients on oral contraceptives as in the control group without hormonal medication. In other words: in this experiment we could not demonstrate a contraceptive effect of the pill by influencing the peritoneal fluid.

References

1. Bouckaert, P. X. J. M., van Wersch, J. W. J. and Schellekens, L. A. (1984). Haemostatic and fibrinolytic properties in the peritoneal fluid in the menstrual cycle. *Br. J. Obstet. Gynaecol.*, **91**, 256
2. Koch, U. J., Hammerstein, J. and Zielske, F. (1977). Der Nachweis von Spermatozoen in der Peritonealflüssigkeit als Parameter der Fertilität. *Arch. Gynaecol.*, **224**, 438
3. Kremer, J. (1965). A simple sperm penetration test. *Int. J. Fertil.*, **10**, 209
4. Roumen, F. J. M. E., Doesburg, W. H. and Rolland, R. (1982). Hormonal patterns in infertile women with a deficient postcoital test. *Fertil. Steril.*, **38**, 42–7

13
Carbohydrate metabolism alterations under monophasic, sequential and triphasic oral contraceptives containing ethinyloestradiol plus levonorgestrel or desogestrel

U. J. GASPARD, M. A. ROMUS AND A. S. LUYCKX

INTRODUCTION

Numerous studies have shown that oral contraceptives affect carbohydrate (CHO) metabolism, and hence may partly lead to atherogenesis and vascular disease. Whereas the oestrogen component of oral contraceptives (OCs) seems to produce few adverse effects on CHO metabolism, 19-norprogestogens have been shown to adversely affect glucose tolerance[1]. One of the possible mechanisms of action of 19-norprogestogens could be related to a reduction in the number and/or affinity of membrane insulin receptors[2].

We investigated carbohydrate metabolism in women receiving OCs containing low doses of 19-norprogestogens, levonorgestrel (LNg) or desogestrel (DOG), a new 3-deoxo 11β-methylene levonorgestrel derivative, in order to compare the potential changes observed in glucose tolerance when using these two progestogens.

SUBJECTS AND METHODS

All women studied ($n = 38$) were healthy volunteers (mean age 22.75 years) within 15% of ideal body weight, who had never used oral contraception previously or had stopped OCs at least 8 weeks prior to the study. In each

Table 1 Oral contraceptives used in this study

Nature of the preparations	Triphasic	Sequential	Monophasic
Trade Names	*Trigynon*	*Ovidol*	*Marvelon*
Components	1. Ethinyloestradiol (EE) 0.03 mg + LNg 0.05 mg (days 1–6)	1. EE 0.05 mg (days 1–7)	EE 0.03 mg + DOG 0.150 mg (days 1–21)
	2. EE 0.04 mg + LNg 0.075 mg (days 7–11)	2. EE 0.05 mg + DOG 0.125 mg (days 8–21)	
	3. EE 0.03 mg + LNg 0.125 mg (days 12–21)		

individual a 3 hour, 75 g oral glucose tolerance test (OGTT) was performed at the end of a spontaneous, control cycle and again at the end of the 6th cycle of OC use. Women were allocated at random to Trigynon ($n = 13$), Ovidol ($n = 11$) or Marvelon ($n = 14$). Composition of the OCs used is given in Table 1.

Fasting blood samples and specimens collected at 30 min intervals during the OGTTs were analysed for blood glucose (BG), blood pyruvate (PYR), plasma immunoreactive insulin (IRI) and plasma immunoreactive glucagon (IRG). Erythrocyte insulin receptors were also measured before and after 6 months of OC use. The methods used are described elsewhere[3].

RESULTS

OGTTs

For each OC used, relative areas under mean BG, PYR, IRI and IRG curves during OGTT (3 hours) obtained during the 6th cycle of treatment have been expressed in per cent change from pretreatment areas under the curves (AUC). Results are shown in Table 2.

Table 2 Relative areas under mean blood glucose, pyruvate, insulin and glucagon curves during OGTT (3 hours)

	Areas (% pretreatment at cycle 6)		
	Triphasic (EE + LNg) Trigynon	Monophasic (EE + DOG) Marvelon	Sequential (EE + DOG) Ovidol
Blood glucose	+12 (%)*	+9	+7
Blood pyruvate	+26†	+2	+20
Plasma insulin	−22*	−24*	−25*
Insulin area/glucose area	−31	−29	−31
Plasma glucagon	+29	+58	+62

*$p < 0.05$
†$p < 0.005$ (difference from pretreatment mean, paired t analysis)

The three groups did not differ significantly as far as BG, PYR, IRI and IRG levels were concerned during the pretreatment cycle. When comparing the three groups after 6 months of treatment (non-paired *t*-test) the AUCs (0–180 min) for BG, IRI, PYR and IRG were not statistically different. However, the AUCs for IRG were distinctly higher under DOG containing OCs than under Trigynon treatment.

Insulin receptors

Erythrocyte insulin receptor levels were in the range of normal premenopausal female controls and were not influenced by OC use (Table 3).

Table 3 Erythrocyte insulin receptors (% of binding)

OCs used	n	Pretreatment cycle	6th cycle of OC use
Triphasic (EE + LNg)	13	8.39 ± 1.19*	8.36 ± 1.38
Monophasic (EE + DOG)	14	7.99 ± 1.33	8.60 ± 1.98
Sequential (EE + DOG)	11	7.85 ± 2.02	7.74 + 1.05

*Mean ± SD. All changes are N.S.

DISCUSSION AND CONCLUSIONS

A slight deterioration of glucose tolerance is observed at 6 months' use of the three OCs, and is somewhat more obvious under Trigynon on the basis of paired *t*-test analysis. However, BG levels never reached pathological levels in any of the volunteers tested. Moreover, no statistical difference concerning glucose tolerance could be delineated between the three groups during the 6th month of treatment (non-paired *t*-test analysis). Blood pyruvate levels fluctuated in the same way as BG levels. Insulin responsiveness was reduced by 20% in all three groups, an observation at variance with other studies[1]. These changes could merely reflect circannual fluctuations in insulin response rather than drug-induced alterations in B-cell responsiveness and/or insulin sensitivity[4]. In the present study, we confirmed in all three groups a decrease by 30% of the insulin area/glucose area ratio, at 6 months of OC use, an observation made previously by Wynn[5]. Moreover, it is noteworthy that IRG was correctly suppressed during OGTT under Trigynon, but not under DOG containing OCs. Altogether, our data indicate that the slight glucose tolerance impairment observed at 6 months of OC use is more clearly discernible under Trigynon than under Marvelon and Ovidol. In our study, glucose tolerance impairment is apparently not correlated with insulin resistance and hyperinsulinism but, in contrast, with decreased insulin secretion. Moreover, a reduction of insulin

79

receptor number or affinity cannot be postulated to explain glucose tolerance deterioration as insulin receptor binding capacity remained stable during OC use in this study.

ACKNOWLEDGEMENTS

We wish to thank Dr Pierre de Meyts (International Institute of Cellular and Molecular Pathology, Catholic University of Louvain, Belgium) who kindly performed the insulin receptor assays.

References

1. Spellacy, W. N. (1982). Carbohydrate metabolism during treatment with estrogen, progestogen and low-dose oral contraceptives. *Am. J. Obstet. Gynecol.*, **142**, 732
2. De Pirro, R., Fiorella, F., Bertoli, A., Greco, A. V. and Lauro, R. (1981). Changes in insulin receptors during oral contraception. *J. Clin. Endocrinol. Metab.*, **52**, 29
3. Luyckx, A. S., Gaspard, U. J., Romus, M. A., De Meyts, P. and Lefebvre, P. J. (1984). Carbohydrate metabolism in women using oral contraceptives containing levonorgestrel or desogestrel. A six month prospective study. (*Fertil. Steril.*, submitted for publication)
4. Reinberg, A., Touitou, Y., Guillemant, S., Levi, S. and Lagoguey, M. (1982). Les rythmes circadiens et circannuels des résultats d'épreuves fonctionnelles en endocrinologie. *Ann. Endocrinol.* (Paris), **43**, 309
5. Wynn, V. (1982). Effect of duration of low-dose oral contraceptive administration on carbohydrate metabolism. *Am. J. Obstet. Gynecol.*, **142**, 739

14
Impact of oral contraceptives upon serum lipoprotein pattern in healthy women

W. MÄRZ, G. ROMBERG, G. GAHN, W. GROß,
H. KUHL AND H.-D. TAUBERT

INTRODUCTION

Epidemiological studies have clearly shown that changes in lipoprotein patterns correlate with the incidence of cardiovascular disease (CVD), in that the risk of myocardial infarction increases when low-density lipoprotein (LDL) and very-low-density lipoproteins (VLDL) are elevated, and high-density lipoproteins (HDL) are lower than normal[1]. The lower susceptibility of women of reproductive age has causally been linked to the lower level of triglycerides (TG) and higher level of HDL as compared to men of equal age. As oestrogens and progestogens, particularly those of the oestrane type, have been recognized as acting differently upon lipoproteins, the former increasing TG and HDL, and the latter having an opposite effect, oral contraceptives (OC) have been implicated as causing an increase of CVD in users[2]. Inasmuch as the present evidence is somewhat contradictory, and it has been shown that various OCs containing different dosages of ethinyl oestradiol (EE) and of levonorgestrel (NG) brought about different effects upon HDL-cholesterol and the HDL-cholesterol to cholesterol ratio, it appears mandatory to examine every new OC with respect to its atherogenic potential. We are reporting here preliminary results of a study comparing the effect of two low-dosed OCs upon lipoprotein patterns in young healthy women.

MATERIALS AND METHODS

Twenty-two healthy female volunteers (aged 24–35 years) with a proven ovulatory cycle participated in the study. None of them had taken any hormonal contraceptive for at least 3 months. Preparation A was a combined, triphasic OC containing 30 μg EE and 50 μg NG (6 days), 40 μg EE and 75 μg NG (5 days), and 30 μg EE and 125 μg NG (10 days; Triquilar). Preparation B contained 30 μg EE and 150 μg desogestrel (DG; Marvelon). Eleven women were randomly assigned to use preparation A for 3 months. This was followed by a wash-out period of 3 months. Thereafter, Preparation B was taken for another 3 months. This sequence was reversed in the remaining 11 volunteers. Fasting-blood samples were obtained at 0800 hours on days 6, 11, 21 and 28 of the (ovulatory) control cycle (C-1) preceding the first treatment cycle. This was repeated during the third treatment cycle (T-1), the third wash-out cycle (C-2), and the third treatment cycle (T-2) after the preparations had been switched.

Cholesterol (Chol) (CHOD-PAP-method, Boehringer Mannheim), triglycerides (TG) (Peridochrom triglycerides, Boehringer Mannheim), and phospholipids (PL) (phospholipid B-test, WAKO fine chemicals Ltd, Osaka) were quantified enzymatically using commercially provided kits. HDL-Cholesterol was determined after selective precipitation of apolipoprotein B containing lipoproteins by an appropriate sodium phosphotungstate/$MgCL_2$ reagent[3]. Quantitative electrophoresis of lipoproteins was performed as described by Wieland et al.[4] Apolipoprotein A-I[5] and apolipoprotein B[6] were determined using Mancini's single radial immunodiffusion technique with the respective monospecific antiserum.

RESULTS

Total lipid levels

The effect of a 3-month course of treatment with the two OCs is depicted in Figure 1. The open bars represent the combined mean values ± SD of the determination of Chol, TG, and PL on days 6, 11, 21 and 28 in 11 volunteers during a control cycle; shaded bars correspond to the respective values recorded during the third month of administration of preparation A (left panel) and preparation B (right panel). There was no discernible effect upon total Chol of either compound as compared to the control cycle. The triphasic preparation increased TG from 93.4 ± 32.1 mg/dl to 111.9 ± 37.6 mg/dl, and the combined preparation brought about a rise from 120.8 ± 46.4 mg/dl to 138.8 ± 53.1 mg/dl. These differences were not statistically significant. Similarly, the observed increases in plasma PL levels (A = + 6%; B = + 10%) were of no significance.

When the data were calculated separately for days 6, 11, 21 and 28 of C-1 and T-1, no differences could be demonstrated.

Lipoprotein pattern

There was a remarkable congruence between the effects of both OCs upon plasma levels of pre-β-lipoprotein-cholesterol, β-lipoprotein-cholesterol, and

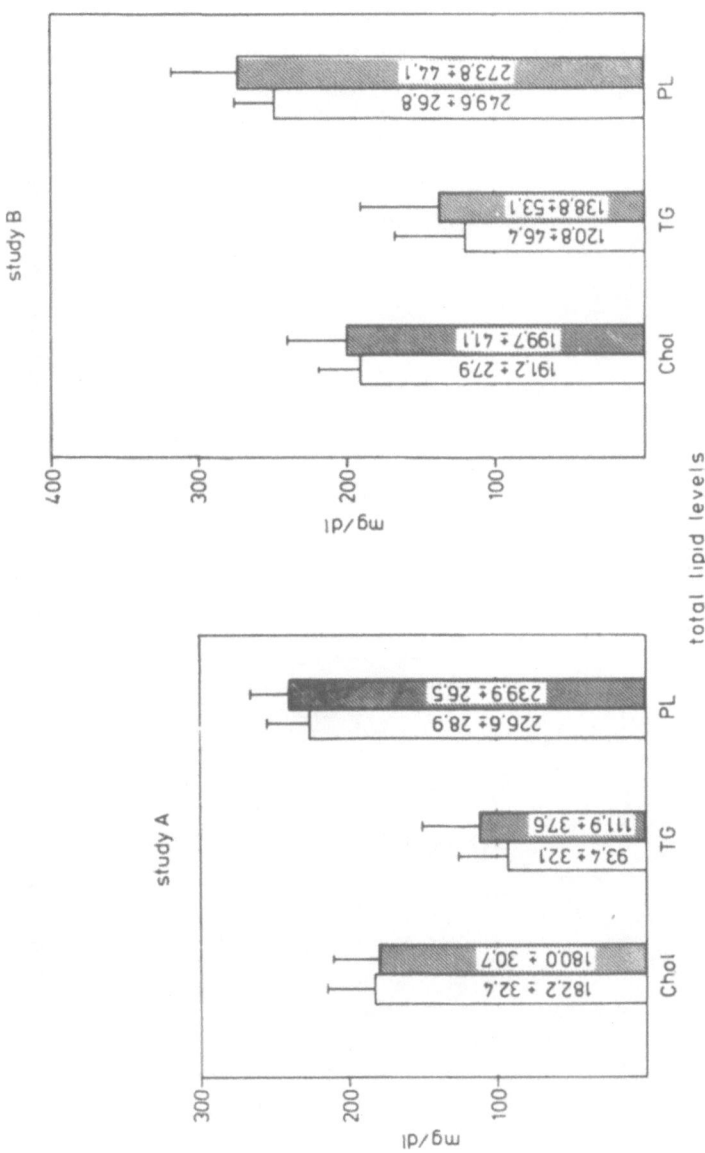

Figure 1 Total lipid levels before and during treatment with a triphasic OC (study A) and a low-dosed combined OC (study B). Open bars: mean ± SD of 4 assays per volunteer (n = 11) in an ovulatory control cycle. Shaded bars: values obtained during the third month of treatment

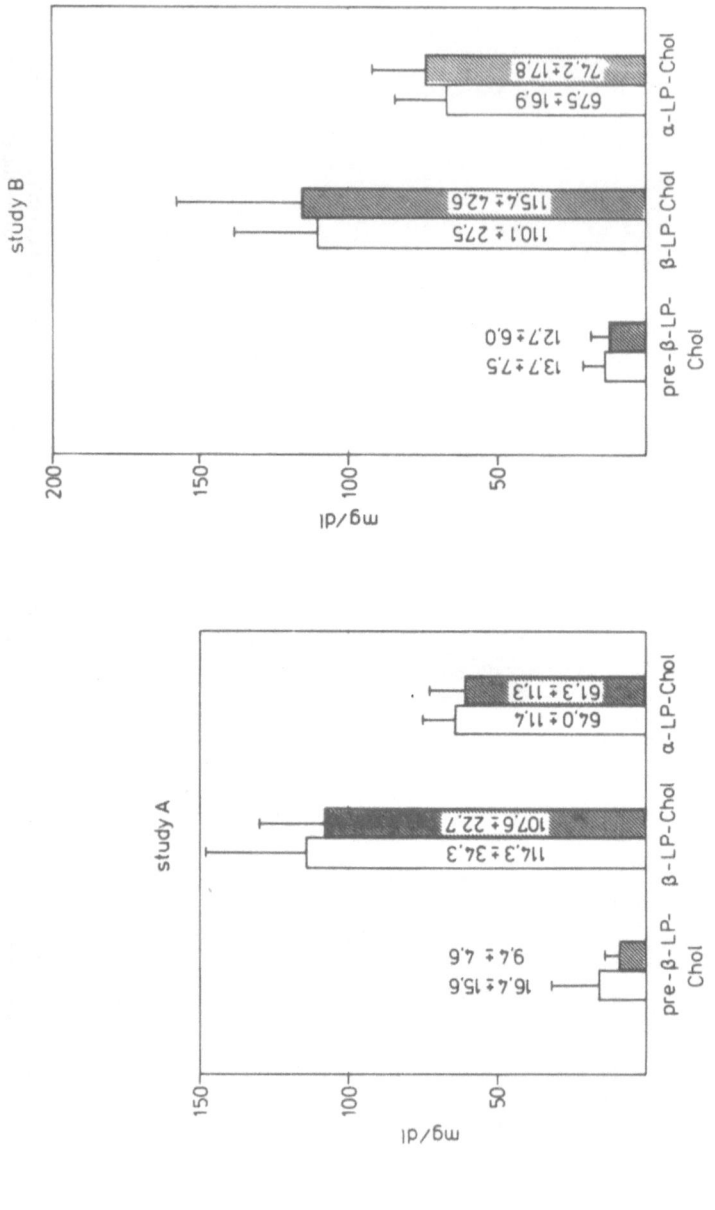

Figure 2 Lipoprotein fractions before and during treatment with a triphasic OC (study A) and a low-dosed combined OC (study B). For details refer to Figure 1 legend

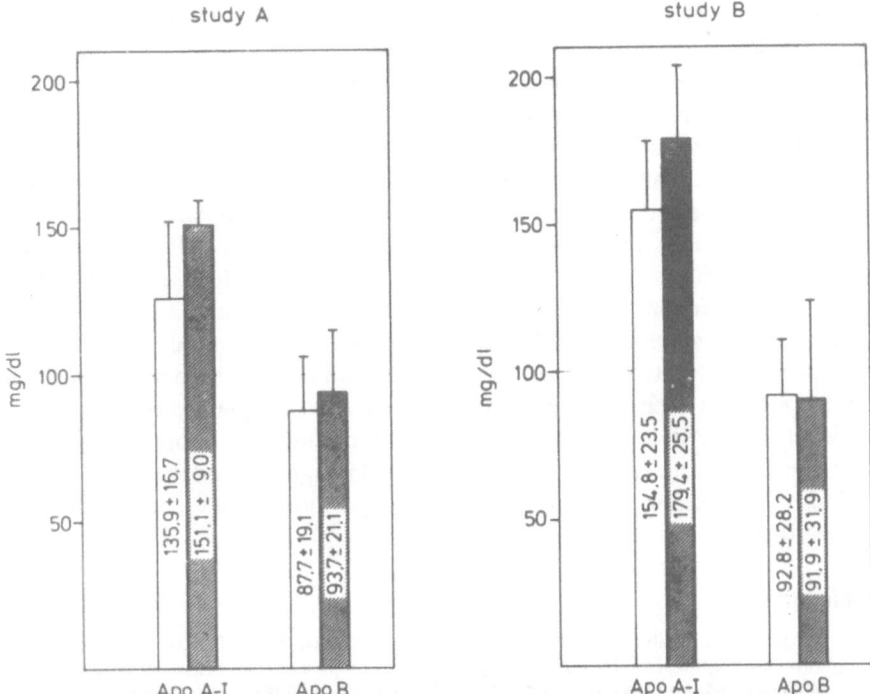

Figure 3 Apolipoprotein A-I and B levels before and during treatment with a triphasic OC (study A) and a low-dosed combined OC (study B). For details refer to legend to Figure 1. The differences between means were of statistical significance ($p < 0.05$; Rank sum test, Mann-Whitney)

α-lipoprotein-cholesterol, in that there was no difference between the mean levels observed during C-1 and T-1 (Figure 2). In addition, no change in HDL-Chol levels could be observed when the sodium phosphotungstate/MgCl$_2$ method was used.

Only apolipoprotein A-I was slightly but significantly increased ($p < 0.01$) by both OCs (A = + 11%; B = + 16%), the increase being in each case of the same order of magnitude (Figure 3).

COMMENT

A final conclusion on the effect of the two low-dose OCs upon the lipoprotein pattern in the plasma of healthy women should not be drawn before the results of the second part of the study have become available. As each treatment period had to be limited to 3 months, changes in TG may escape detection, as this might not become noticeable before 3–6 months of treatment, as compared to a reduction in HDL which becomes demonstrable within 1 month[7]. Since the data of the first treatment period are more or less consistent with each other, it does not appear likely that major changes will be noted after the cross-over.

Whereas HDL-cholesterol levels were not affected by either OC a slight but significant increase of apolipoprotein A-I could be shown as compared to the control cycle. This reflects a change in the composition of HDL which may be in part due to the relatively greater decrease of chol-rich HDL_2 density class than that of HDL_3[8]. The principle abnormality of HDL in CVD appears to be a relative decrease in the molar concentration of HDL_2 accompanied by a decrease in total HDL-chol[8, 9]. Since we did not find any change in the HDL-chol concentrations, it remains to be shown whether the observed decrease in the HDL-chol/apolipoprotein A-I ratio reflects an atherogenic constellation.

It should be emphasized that the results of this study can only be considered as being representative for healthy females devoid of any disorder of lipoprotein metabolism, as such a disorder may be intensified by the use of OCs[10].

We conclude that Triquilar and Marvelon do not alter lipoprotein patterns in women, without risk factors, in a detrimental manner, and that both preparations do not differ with respect to that, even though they contain different progestogens.

References

1. Gordon, T., Castelli, W. P., Hjortland, M. C. and Kannel, W. B. (1977). The prediction of coronary heart disease by high density and other lipoproteins: an historical perspective. In Rifkind, B. M. and Levy R. I. (eds.) *Hyperlipidema* p. 71. (New York: Grune and Stratton)
2. Heiss, G., Ramir, I., Davis, C. E., Tyroler, H. A., Rifkind, B. M., Schonfeld, G., Jacobs, D. and Rantz, I. D. (1980). Lipoprotein-cholesterol distributions in selected North American populations: the Lipids Research Clinics Programme prevalence study. *Circulation*, 61, 302
3. Assmann, G., Schriewer, H. and Funke, H. (1981). Zur Richtigkeit der HDL-Cholesteron and HDL-Apolipoprotein A-I Bestimmung nach Phosphwolframsäure/MgCl₂-Präzipitation Apolipoprotein B-haltiger Lipoproteine. *J. Clin. Chem. Biochem.*, 19, 273
4. Wieland, H., Niazi, M., Bartholomé, M. and Seidel, D. (1980). Eine neue Methode zur Messung von Plasmalipoproteinen. *Ärztl. Lab.*, 26, 257.
5. Cheung, M. D. and Albers, J. J. (1977). The measurement of apolipoprotein A-I and A-II levels in men and women by immunoassay. *J. Clin. Invest.*, 60, 43
6. Heuck, C. C., Oster, P., Rapp, W. and Schlierf, G. (1977). Differentialdiagnostik der Hyperlipoproteinämien mit Hilfe der Bestimmung von Apolipoprotein B. *Ärztl. Lab.*, 23, 143
7. Larsson-Cohn, U., Fåhraeus, L., Wallentin, L. and Zador, G. (1981). Lipoprotein changes may be minimized by proper composition of a combined oral contraceptive. *Fertil. Steril.*, 35, 172
8. Albers, J. J., Cheung, M. C. and Hazzard, W. R. (1978). High-density lipoproteins in myocardial infarction survivors. *Metab. Clin. Exp.*, 27, 479
9. Hammet, F., Saltissi, S., Miller, N., Rao, S., Van-Zeller, H., Coltart, J. and Lewis, B. (1979). Relationship of coronary atherosclerosis to plasma lipoproteins. *Circulation*, 60, 11
10. Zorilla, E., Hulse, M., Hernandez, A. and Gehrberg, H. (1968). Severe endogenous triglyceridemia during treatment with estrogen and oral contraceptives. *J. Clin. Endocrinol. Metab.*, 28, 576

15
Androgenic action of progestins used in oral contraceptives

J. SPONA

INTRODUCTION

Concomitant androgenic and oestrogenic potencies of progestational components of oral contraceptives are well documented by pharmacological studies in animals and man[1,2]. Androgen related side-effects are unwanted and should be kept as small as possible. Desogestrel[3] and its biologically active metabolite 3-keto-desogestrel (13-ethyl-11-methylene-18,19-dinor-17α-pregn-4-en-20-yn-17-ol-3-one), respectively, were reported to lack androgenicity in the dose used for oral contraception[4]. Reduced androgenic properties of 3-keto-desogestrel compared with levonorgestrel and other compounds were explained on grounds of receptor studies[5].

The aim of the present investigation was to study in detail the receptor interactions of various progestagens, and to correlate receptor data with biological activity with respect to androgen effects in a model system.

MATERIALS AND METHODS

Mouse kidney cytosol was used as the model system to test for relative binding affinities (RBA) of 3-keto-desogestrel, levonorgestrel, dihydrotestosterone, 17α-propylmesterolone, cyproterone acetate and progesterone. Determination of RBA was carried out essentially as previously described[6]. Briefly, cytosol samples were incubated with 120 000 cpm [³H]R1881 (specific activity 81 Ci/mmol) in the presence of 0–10 000 nmol/l of the progestagen to be tested. Unlabelled R1881 was used as the reference substance to determine RBA, which was calculated by computer programs run on a PDP 11/34 DEC datasystem

(Digital Equipment Corporation, Maynard, MA, USA). RBA was calculated by dividing the concentration of R1881 which displaces 50% of [^{3}H]R1881 by the 50% intercept concentration of the progestagen tested. Incubations were carried out in triplicate and RBA data were derived from seven different experiments. Statistical evaluation of data was performed by the Student t-test.

Stimulation of β-glucuronidase activity was used as the parameter to test various steroids for androgenicity. Progestins were subcutaneously applied to adult female mice at 0.05, 0.5 and 1.5 mg daily dose for 7 days. Steroids were dissolved in sesame oil with 10% ethyl alcohol. Control groups were injected with the vehicle only. Each treatment group consisted of five animals. Mice were sacrificed 4 h after the last application. β-glucuronidase activity was determined by methods previously published[7]. Results are expressed as per cent enzyme activity of control groups. Data are means ± SD of enzyme activities in 10 kidneys of each group.

RESULTS

Significantly greater affinity ($p < 0.02$) of 3-keto-desogestrel than of levonorgestrel for the androgen-receptor was noted (Figure 1). Progesterone exhibited only residual affinity for mouse kidney cytosolic androgen-receptor. Greatest affinity was noted for dihydrotestosterone. Cyproterone acetate and 17α-propylmesterolone had an affinity similar to that of levonorgestrel.

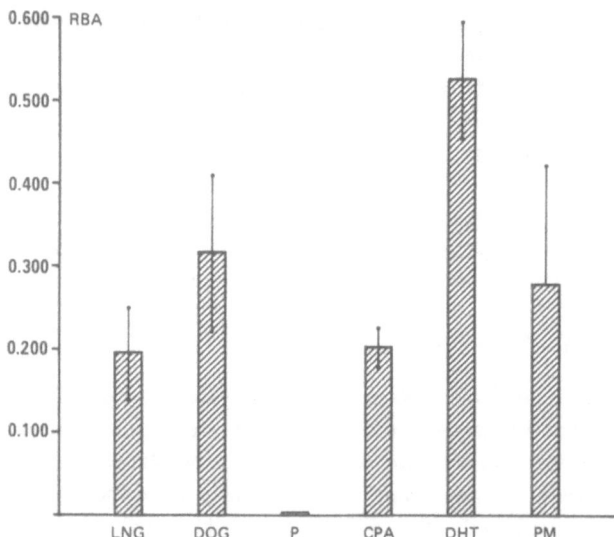

Figure 1 Relative binding affinity (RBA) of levonorgestrel (LNG), 3-keto-desogestrel (DOG), progesterone (P), cyproterone acetate (CPA), dihydrotestosterone (DHT) and 17α-propyl-mesterolone (PM)

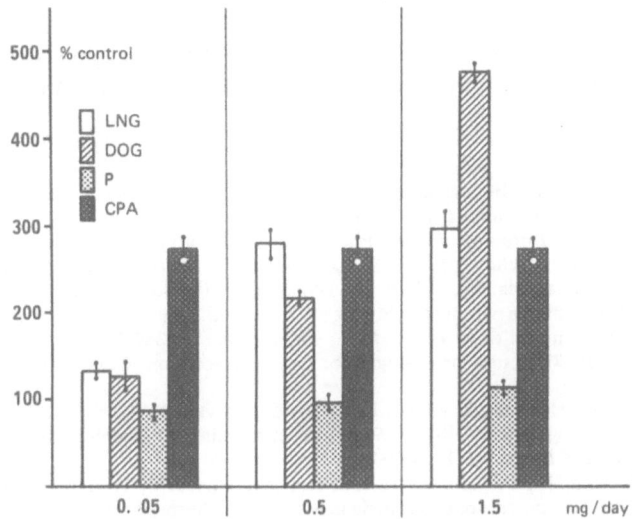

Figure 2 β-Glucuronidase activity stimulated by various progestins over vehicle treated animals (100%). Key: as Figure 1

Experiments on β-glucuronidase activity revealed no significant differences between levonorgestrel and 3-keto-desogestrel at the lower doses, but significantly greater ($p < 0.005$) enzyme stimulation at the 1.5 mg dose (Figure 2). Progesterone did not stimulate enzyme activity. Cyproterone acetate and 17α-propylmesterolone, respectively, exhibited dose-independent stimulation of β-glucuronidase to some 300% of controls.

DISCUSSION

The most interesting result of the present investigation was the observation that 3-keto-desogestrel exhibited significantly greater affinity than levonorgestrel for the mouse kidney cytosol receptor (Figure 1). These data differ from those of previous reports[2]. These studies[2] were done in only one single experiment. Opposite results[2] from those of the present investigation led to the conclusion that 3-keto-desogestrel was less androgenic than levonorgestrel. But, present data corroborate a previous report[8] where prostate cytosol was used as the receptor source.

In addition, androgenic potency as estimated by β-glucuronidase activity showed 3-keto-desogestrel to be more androgenic at higher dose levels (Figure 2). Present data and clinical studies[9] combine to suggest that androgen related side-effects should occur more frequently when desogestrel is used in oral contraceptives.

ACKNOWLEDGEMENTS

The expert technical assistance of E. Zatlasch is greatly appreciated. We gratefully acknowledge the secretarial work provided by J. Reinauer.

References

1. Brotherton, J. (1976). Biological assessment. In Brotherton, J. (ed.) *Sexhormone pharmacology*. pp. 43–78. (London and New York: Academic Press)
2. Briggs, M. H. and Briggs, M. (1976). Pharmacology. In Briggs, M. H. and Briggs, M. (eds.) *Biochemical Contraception*. pp. 69–72. (London and New York: Academic Press)
3. Viinikka, L., Ylikorkala, O., Vihko, R., Wijnand, H. P., Booij, M. and van der Venn, F. (1979). Metabolism of a new synthetic progestagen, ORG.2969, in female volunteers. Pharmacokinetics after an oral dose. *Eur. J. Clin., Pharmacol.*, **15**, 349–55
4. De Jager, E. (1982). A new progestagen for oral contraception. *Contracept. Deliv. Syst.*, **3**, 11–15
5. Bergink, E. W., Hamburger, A. D., De Jager, E. and van der Vies, J. (1981). Binding of a contraceptive progestagen ORG 2969 and its metabolites to receptor proteins and human SHBG. *J. Steroid Biochem.*, **14**, 175–7
6. Spona, K., Ulm, R., Bieglmayer, C. and Husslein, P. (1979). Hormone serum levels and hormone receptor contents of endometria in women with normal menstrual cycles and patients bearing endometrial carcinoma. *Gynecol. Obstet. Invest.*, **10**, 71–80
7. Fishman, W. H. (1974). β-Glucuronidase. In Bergmeyer, H. U. (ed.) *Methoden der enzymatische Analyse*, Band 1, 3. Auflage pp. 964–79. (Weinheim/Bergstr: Verlag Chemie)
8. Gang, S., Anderson, K. M. and Liao, S. (1969). Receptor proteins for androgens. On the role of specific proteins in selective retention for 17β-hydroxy-5α-androstan-e-one by rat ventral prostate *in vivo* and *in vitro*. *J. Biol. Chem.*, **244**, 6548–91
9. Lachnit-Fixson, U. (1983). Comparison between Marvelon(®) and Triquilar(®). In Harrison, R. H., Bonnar, J. and Thompson, W. (eds.) *Fertility and Sterility*. p. 595. (Lancaster: MTP Press)

16
Triquilar: a low-dose triphasic oral contraceptive

G. LADA AND R. GIMES

INTRODUCTION

With the application of synthetic gestogens and oestrogens first in combined, later in normophasic sequential form a secure contraceptive method was developed which has been used all over the world. As in any other medical treatment this method also has its side effects; e.g. influencing metabolism and blood clotting. Therefore, the aim is to create the most efficient medical effect with the least possible side-effects. There are two ways to obtain this result, one is to reduce the contraceptive hormones to the lowest effective dose, the other being to administer it in doses being close to the physiological level. With these aims in mind we have conducted a clinical trial with a triphasic contraceptive named Triquilar (Schering).

MATERIALS AND METHODS

Figure 1 shows the composition of Triquilar and the timing of administration of the individual components. The dosage regimen starts on day 5 of the cycle with tablets having an excessive oestrogen level. From day 12 the components are nearly balanced, and during the last 10 days of treatment the patients are given tablets containing more gestogens. At the end of the treatment there is a pause of 7 days.

Fifty healthy, normotensive women were given Triquilar; the results studied were obtained from 1800 menstrual cycles. Twenty-three of our patients had never taken contraceptives before, 20 of them biphasic ones and seven had used combined pills. Twenty-one of the patients were nulliparous.

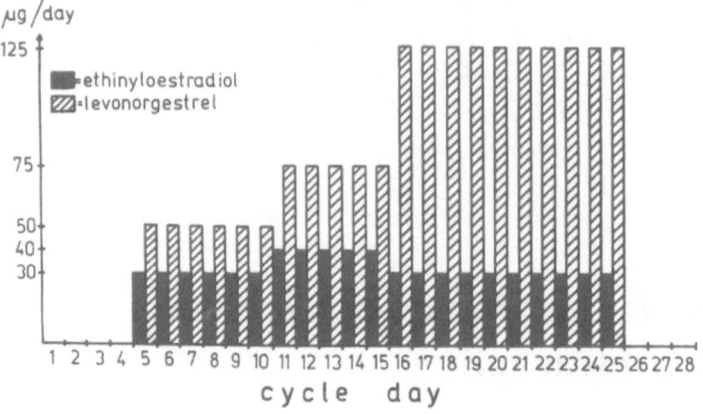

Figure 1 Composition of Triquilar and timing of administration of the individual components

Table 1 Frequency of tests during the administration of Triquilar

Duration of treatment	Routine gynecology	Colpo-cytology	Blood pressure	Body weight	Laboratory	Onco-cytology
before	↓	↓	↓	↓	↓	↓
cycle 1			↓	↓		
2	↓	↓	↓	↓		
3			↓	↓	↓	
4	↓	↓	↓	↓		
5			↓	↓		
6	↓	↓	↓	↓		
7			↓	↓		
8	↓	↓	↓	↓		
9			↓	↓		
10	↓	↓	↓	↓		
11			↓	↓		
12	↓	↓	↓	↓	↓	↓
24	↓	↓	↓	↓	↓	↓
36	↓	↓	↓	↓	↓	↓

Table 1 shows the tests we performed during the treatment. Routine gynaeco-logical and colpocytological examinations were performed on every patient every second month in the first year, and later at yearly intervals. Blood pressure and body weight were checked monthly. We made oncocytological tests at the beginning of the trial and again yearly. We investigated liver function and lipid metabolism, measuring the level of serum bilirubin, total protein, albumin, cholesterol, triglycerides, HDL- and LDL-cholesterol and GOT, GPT, AP activity at the start, in the third month and later yearly.

RESULTS

During the Triquilar administration in 1800 cycles no pregnancy occurred. Table 2 shows the side-effects. Two women complained of nausea, but only during the first two cycles. Two women mentioned breast tension, they had taken biphasic oral contraceptives earlier with the same side-effect. Two of the patients complained about dysmenorrhoea in the first cycle and four women reported their former dysmenorrhoea had ceased. One of the patients reported a temporary decrease of libido and another had an increased libido. Irregular bleeding symptoms, frequently appearing while taking oral contraceptives,

Table 2 Side-effects

Type	No of women	Remarks
Nausea	2	During the first two cycles
Breast tension	2	Also with other kind of pills
Dysmenorrhoea	2	In the first cycle
Decreased libido	1	Temporary
Increased libido	1	Temporary
Breakthrough bleeding	3	In cycle 2, 4, 28
Spotting	3	In cycle 1, 3, 3–6
Mycotic vaginal infection	4	After one treatment cured
Thromboembolic complications	–	—

occurred in three cases, spotting appeared in another three cases. After stopping the medication, withdrawal bleeding occurs on day 2 or 3. The duration and intensity of bleeding in most cases was the same as usual. Mycotic vaginal infection occurred in four cases, but it was cured during the first series of treatment. Thromboembolic complications did not occur during the period of observation. No pathological changes have been found by routine gynaecological and oncocytological examinations. No significant change in blood pressure could be found during the trial in previously normotensive women. The low increase of the body weight is very favourable. Only two of the patients put on 4 kg and six of them 2 kg during the treatment. Two obese patients lost body weight after their oligomenorrhoea had been cured with the pills. The colpocytological examinations were made on stained or fresh smears. The picture varies depending on the exogene hormone intake during the physiological cycle in each case, and no atrophic signs ever appeared. This is very important, because in the course of administering combined contraceptives, paralleled with the time factor, atrophy does occur. The laboratory values (Figure 2) were carefully examined and revealed smaller fluctuations, however, these proved to be not significant even in relation to lipid metabolism.

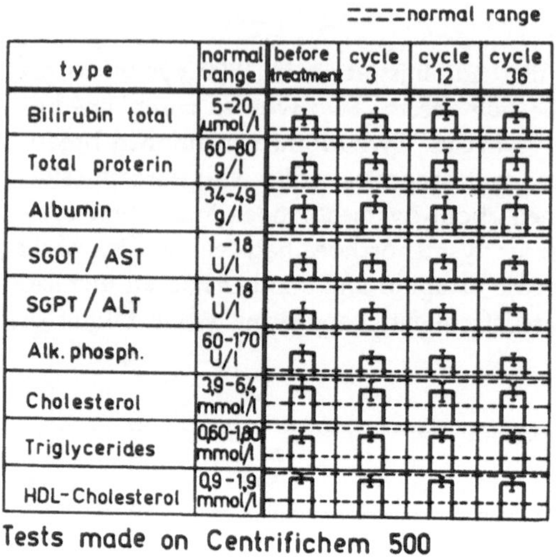

====normal range

type	normal range	before treatment	cycle 3	cycle 12	cycle 36
Bilirubin total	5-20 μmol/l				
Total proterin	60-80 g/l				
Albumin	34-49 g/l				
SGOT / AST	1-18 U/l				
SGPT / ALT	1-18 U/l				
Alk. phosph.	60-170 U/l				
Cholesterol	3,9-6,4 mmol/l				
Triglycerides	0,60-1,80 mmol/l				
HDL-Cholesterol	0,9-1,9 mmol/l				

Tests made on Centrifichem 500

Figure 2   Laboratory tests

DISCUSSION

Table 3 shows the advantages of Triquilar. The great advantage of this pill is that the endometrium is built up during each cycle. Other advantageous changes appear on the vaginal epithelium because of the oestrogen-dominant dose administered at the beginning of the cycle, this is shown by the colpocytological picture. We have to emphasize the fact that nobody had to stop taking the pill because of side-effects. This triphasic contraceptive can be also administered to juveniles. There is no need to consider the possibility that hormonal contraceptives with their atrophic effect may steadily influence the young body. Although the pill gives perfect contraception with oestrogen dominance at the beginning of the cycle it does not cause further atrophy of hypoplastic genital organs, on the contrary, it corrects them.

Table 3   Advantage of Triquilar

1. Low dose
2. New administration scheme
3. Builds up the endometrium
4. Builds up the vaginal epithelium
5. Decreased side-effects
6. Suitable for juveniles

SUMMARY

On the basis of our studies in 1800 cycles we tested a new triphasic oral contraceptive. We found only few, acceptable side-effects. The cytological signs show that the contraceptive builds up the menstrual cycle in a satisfactory way.

Laboratory tests revealed that the new pill does not cause any pathological changes either in blood clotting or in metabolism. Suitable administration of synthetic oestrogens and gestogens gave an optimal build-up of endometrium with the minimal possible doses. The introduction of triphasic low-dose pills should lead to the further development of oral contraceptives.

References

1. Dombrowicz, N. and Van de Walle, J. (1979). Clinical, histological and stereo-morphometric study of a new normophasic oral contraceptives: fysioquens. *IX. World Congress Gynecology and Obstetrics*. Abstract 339, Tokyo
2. Elstein, M. (1978). Studies on low dose oral contraceptives: plasma hormone changes in relation to deliberate pill ("Microgynon 30") omission. *V. European Congress on Sterility and Fertility*. Abstract 239, Venice
3. Gimes R. and Csömör S. (1980). Háromfázisu orális fogamzásgátló alkalmazásával szerzett tapasztalataink. *Magyar Nőorv. L.*, **43**, 501
4. Gimes, R., Horn, B. and Tóth, F. (1969). Sequential jellegü norsteroid (Ovanon) therápiás alkalmazása ovarialis dysfunctiok esetében. *Magyar Nőorv. L.*, **32**, 317
5. Gimes, R. and Tóth, F. (1969). Untersuchungen zur Frage des Rebound Effectes nach Anwendung der Ovanons (Organon). *Deutsch. Med. J.*, **20**, 718
6. Gimes, R. and Tóth, F. (1971). Colpocytological findings in low dose Norsteroid (Lynestrenol) treatment. *4th International Congress of Cytology*. Abstract 142, London
7. Greenblatt, R. B. (1980). A retrospective view of oral contraceptives. In Greenblatt R. B. (ed.) *The Development of a New Triphasic Oral Contraceptive*. p. 1. (Lancaster: MTP Press)
8. Greenblatt, R. B. (ed.) (1980). *The Development of a New Triphasic Oral Contraceptive*. (Lancaster: MTP Press)
9. Haller, J. (1971). Ovulationshemmung durch Hormone. (Stuttgart: G. Thieme Verlag)
10. Hamvas, F., Kovács, I., Gimes, R. and Csömör, S. (1978). Noretiszteron (Norcolut) alkalmazásával szerzett tapasztalataink. *Gyógyszereink*, **28**, 251
11. Hines, D. C. and Goldzieher, J. (1968). Large-scale study of an oral contraceptive. *Fertil. Steril.*, **19**, 841
12. Loraine, J., Bell, E. T., Harkness, R. A., Mears, E. and Jackson, M. (1965). Hormone excretion patterns during and after the longterm administration of oral contraceptives. *Acta Endocrinol.*, **50**, 15
13. Lachnit-Fixson, U. (1980). The rational for a new triphasic contraceptive. In Greenblatt, R. B. (ed.) *The Development of a New Triphasic Oral Contraceptive*. p. 23. (Lancaster: MTP Press)
14. Robertson, S., Birrel, W. and Grant, A. (1978). Defective ovulation – Before and after the era of the contraceptive pills. A study of 9819 patients. *V. European Congress on Sterility and Fertility*. Abstract 237, Venice
15. Schellen, T. and Dufais, L. J. (1978). "Sub-50" pills: the new trend in oral contraception. *V. European Congress in Sterility and Fertility*. Abstract 240, Venice
16. Seregély, Gy. (1976). Fogamzásgátlás. *Budapest Medicina Könyvkiadó*, 317
17. Seregély, Gy. (1979). Néhány adat és szempont a gyógyszerinteractiok és orális kontraceptivumok összefüggéséhez. *Gyógyszereink*, **29**, 258
18. Taymor, M. L. and Green, T. H. (1975). *Progress in Gynecology*. (New York: Grune and Stratton)
19. Tóth, F., Gimes, R. and Csömör, S. (1968). Histokémiai vizsgálatok Orgametrillel és Lindiolsequentiallal kezelt asszonyok endometriumán. *Magyar Nőorv. L.*, **31**, 325
20. Tóth, F., Gimes, R. and Horn, B. (1972). Klinikai vizsgálatok kis dosisu contraceptivumokkal. *Magyar Nőorv. L.*, **35**, 530
21. Tóth, F., Gimes, R., Horn, B. and Kerényi, T. (1972). Az endometrium histochemiai és ultrastructurális vizsgálata kis dosisu kontraceptivumok adagolása során. *Magyar Nőorv. L.*, **35**, 123

22. Tóth, F., Kerényi, T. and Gimes, R. (1974). Az endometrium histochemiai és elektron-mikroszkópos vizsgálata kombinált és sequential kontraceptiv kezelés alatt. Korányi Társ. Tud. Ülései XIII., Budapest, Akadémiai Kiadó, 91, 104
23. Villedieu, P. (1979). Oral contraceptives. *IX. World Congress on Gynecology, and Obstetrics.* Abstract 345, Tokyo
24. Virginia, Uptun, G. (1980). The normal menstrual cycle and oral contraceptives. The physiological basis for a triphasic approach. In Greenblatt, R. B. (ed.) *The Development of a New Triphasic Oral Contraceptive.* p. 31. (Lancaster: MTP Press)

17
Possible protection from breast cancer with long-term oral contraceptive use

R. D. GAMBRELL, Jr. AND R. C. MAIER

INTRODUCTION

Because of the uncertain role of sex steroids in breast cancer, speculation has arisen that any carcinogenic potential of birth control pills might not be detectable for 10 years or more. It was estimated that 10 000 000 women in the United States were using oral contraceptives in the mid-1970s, although that number had decreased by the early 1980s. Breast cancer is not only the most frequent malignancy in women (27% of all cancers), but is also the leading cause of death from cancer in females (19% of all cancer deaths) in the US. As part of the continuing studies on the relationship of hormones to cancer at Wilford Hall USAF Medical Center[1], the cases of breast cancer during the past 7 years in premenopausal women comprise the basis for this report.

MATERIALS AND METHODS

Patients with breast cancer were identified from the tumour registry. Once a patient is entered into this registry, outpatient records are coded so that copies of all visits are forwarded for inclusion. Oral contraceptive use data was available for the 7 years from 1975–1981, obtained from computerized pharmacy records, and is based upon the number of birth control pills stocked and dispensed to patients. Statistical analysis of the data was performed by the Systems and Computer Services, Medical College of Georgia, using the test for significance of differences between 2 proportions.

RESULTS

There were 63 patients with breast cancer diagnosed from our clinic population from 1975–1981. A negative history of hormone usage was obtained from 39 of these 63 women (61.9%). There were 24 women in this group who either were using oral contraceptives when the mammary malignancy was detected or gave a past history of birth control pill use. Duration of use varied from 3 months to 15 years, and 19 patients had discontinued use from 3 months to 15 years prior to detection of the breast cancer. The number of patients using oral contraceptives during the 7 years are as follows: 1975, 8693; 1976, 7566; 1977, 6376; 1978, 7236; 1979, 6848; 1980, 6377; 1981, 5563. There was a trend away from prescribing pills with a high oestrogen content ($>50\,\mu g$) towards those containing smaller amounts of oestrogen ($50\,\mu g$ or less). During the 7 years there was a decline in oral contraceptive use by 26%, from 8693 users in 1975 to 5563 users during 1981, although clinic populations slightly increased.

Only the incidence of breast cancer among current oral contraceptive users could be calculated, since it is unknown how many patients from our clinic population had a past history of birth control pill usage. There were five women using oral contraceptives at the time breast cancer was diagnosed during 48 659 patient-years of observation, giving an annual incidence rate of $10.3:100\,000$ women (Table 1). Five other patients had used birth control pills until 3–14

Table 1 Incidence of breast cancer in oral contraceptive users: 1975–1981

Oral contraceptive use	Patient years of observation	Mean age (range)	Patients with cancer	Incidence (per 100 000)
Current use	48 659	36.6 (35–39)	5	10.3*
Use within 1 year	>48 659	36.6 (31–44)	10	<20.6
Any past history	>48 659	40.9 (31–53)	24	<49.3
Third National Cancer Survey (1975)		(35–39)		53.3
NCI SEER (1980)		(35–39)		57.3

*$p \leqslant 0.05$

months before detection of breast cancer. Including these five patients, the incidence of mammary malignancy was less than $20.6:100\,000$ women per year. Including all 24 women with a history of oral contraceptive use, the incidence of breast cancer was less than $49.3:100\,000$. All three of these incidence rates are lower than the expected incidence in this age group, $53.3:100\,000$, according to the Third National Cancer Survey, which was conducted just prior to our study. These incidence rates are also lower than that of the National Cancer Institute SEER data ($57.3:100\,000$) which was reported toward the end of our study.

DISCUSSION

The role of oral contraceptives as a possible cause of breast carcinoma has been of concern for many years. At Wilford Hall USAF Medical Center the incidence of breast cancer among oral contraceptive users (10.3:100 000) is significantly lower ($p \leqslant 0.05$) than expected, according to both the Third National Cancer Survey (53.3:100 000) and the National Cancer Institute SEER data (57.2:100 000). Even including all the 'ever' birth control pill users, the annual incidence rate was less than 49.3:100 000, which is still lower than that expected from both of the national surveys. Recognizing the limitations of this study, it is apparent that the incidence of breast cancer is decreased in oral contraceptive users.

Several epidemiologic studies have either not found any increased risk of breast cancer in anovulant users or lower rates of malignancy in those taking birth control pills[2-4]. In the Walnut Creek study, the incidence of breast cancer in the 'ever' oral contraceptive users, ages 18–39, was 25:100 000 compared to 55:100 000 in the 'never' users (RR = 0.5)[2]. At all ages, including women to age 64, the incidence of mammary malignancy was 131:100 000 in the 'ever' users and 114:100 000 in the 'never' users (RR = 1.2); however, the difference was not statistically significant. In the Royal College of General Practitioners study, the incidence of mammary malignancy was 47:100 000 in the 'ever' users compared to 39:100 000 in the controls (RR = 1.2)[3]. In the recent Centers for Disease Control Cancer and Steroid Hormone Study, the RR for 'ever' users was 0.9, and women whose first use was more than 15 years ago and who had used oral contraceptives for 11 years or more had a RR of 0.8. It is unfortunate that none of the epidemiologic studies separated their 'ever' users into current users and past users, for if they had they might have obtained a decreased risk of breast cancer in current oral contraceptive users, similar to the findings in our study.

Most studies list pregnancy, lactation and increased parity as potentially protective conditions for breast cancer. Oral contraceptives, by simulating pregnancy, especially with longterm usage to simulate increasing parity, may exert a protective mechanism from subsequent carcinoma of the breast.

References

1. Gambrell, R. D., Jr., Massey, F. M., Castaneda, T. A. et al. (1979). Breast cancer and oral contraceptive therapy in premenopausal women. J. Reprod. Med., 23, 265
2. Ramcharan, S., Pellegrin, F. A., Ray, R. et al. (1981). The Walnut Creek Contraceptive Drug Study: A Prospective Study of the Side Effects of Oral Contraceptives. Vol. III. (Bethesda, Maryland, USA: Dept. Health and Human Services (NIH))
3. Kay, C. (1981). Breast cancer and oral contraceptives: findings in Royal College of General Practitioners' study. Br. Med. J., 282, 2089
4. Centers for Disease Control Cancer and Steroid Hormone Study. (1983). Long-term oral contraceptive use and the risk of breast cancer. J. Am. Med. Assoc., 249, 1591

18
The effects of active immunization of marmoset monkeys against the beta subunit of ovine luteinizing hormone (oLH Beta)

P. G. SPINOLA, E. M. COUTINHO, V. DOURADO AND R. B. THAU

INTRODUCTION

Chorionic gonadotrophin (CG) is probably a major luteotrophic stimulus of early pregnancy in primates. CG, a product of the implanting trophoblast, is believed to be essential for the ovarian progesterone production which is necessary for normal implantation and for pregnancy maintenance.

Active immunization against CG is a potential method of fertility control[1-3]. The most likely mechanism of action is that the circulating antibodies bind the CG released by the implanting embryo, thereby preventing its stimulating effect on luteal steroidogenesis.

The beta subunit of ovine luteinizing hormone (oLH Beta) is a good possibility for an effective antigen. It has been shown[4] to neutralize the biological activity of CG and to cross-react with LH in the rhesus monkey, thereby sufficiently decreasing progesterone production but without preventing ovulation and regular menstrual cycles. Circulating antibodies to oLH Beta reduced fertility drastically. We believe that active immunization with oLH Beta has the potential to be equally effective in other primates, such as the marmoset and the human.

MATERIALS AND METHODS

Adult marmoset monkeys (*Callithrix jacchus*) were purchased from local dealers and quarantined for 4 months before being used experimentally. They were housed in stable male–female individual pairs in cages of $50 \times 55 \times 75$ cm containing a nest box and perches. The animals were provided with water *ad libitum*, fed with fresh fruits and supplemented with a commercial diet and vitamin C.

Blood was drawn from the femoral vein with a heparinized 1 ml syringe between 0900 and 1200 hours, and the plasma separated by centrifugation and stored at $-20\,°C$ until assayed.

Plasma levels of progesterone were determined by RIA in two complete cycles and weekly thereafter, using the protocol recommended by the WHO Programme for the provision of matched assays and reagents for the radio-immunoassay of hormones in reproductive physiology.

Eight female marmosets were actively immunized with oLH Beta. oLH Beta (S742AP) was a gift from Dr M. R. Sairam, Montreal. 50 μg of oLH Beta was dissolved in 250 μl of saline and emulsified with an equal volume of Freund's complete adjuvant. Multiple sites in the axillary region were injected subcutaneously on day 0 and 3 weeks later. Blood samples were drawn weekly for 8 weeks after immunization.

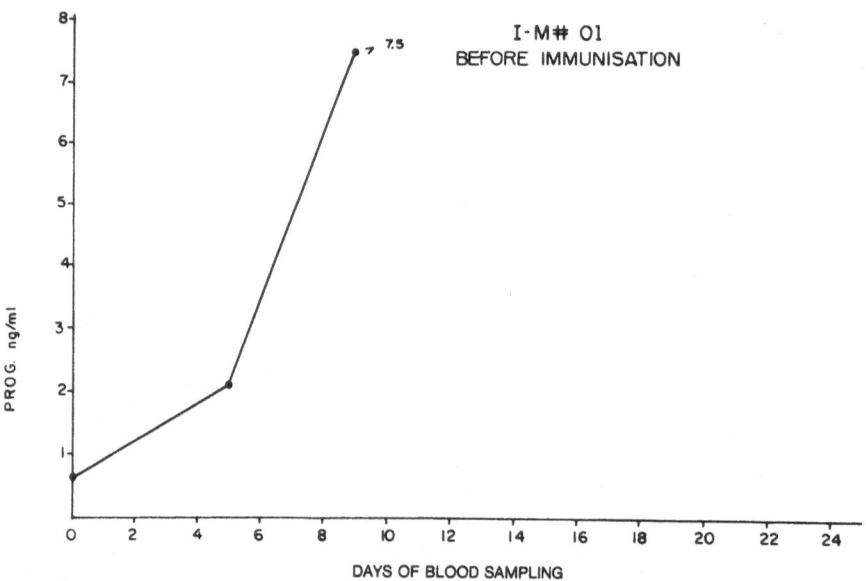

Figure 1 Progesterone levels in the peripheral plasma of non-immunized marmoset monkeys

RESULTS

The results from eight treated animals immunized against oLH Beta showed that in the first control cycle before immunization only three out of eight were ovulating or pregnant (progesterone levels > 7.5 ng/ml) (Figure 1). In the other five animals ovulation did not occur as the progesterone levels were below 3.0 ng/ml (Figure 2). In the second control cycle before immunization all animals showed progesterone levels above 7.5 ng/ml suggesting a normal corpus luteum function or pregnancy (Figure 3).

After immunization five out of eight animals retained plasma progesterone levels above 15 ng/ml (Figure 4), and it may be that no immediate adverse effects occurred in these animals. In the other three animals the plasma progesterone levels were below 3.0 ng/ml (Figure 5), indicating interruption of pregnancy or impaired corpus luteum function.

Two animals immunized in late pregnancy, as judged by abdominal palpation during the immunization procedure, delivered normal live twins.

One abortion was recorded after immunization as the day on which blood was first found on the perches or exuding from the vulva.

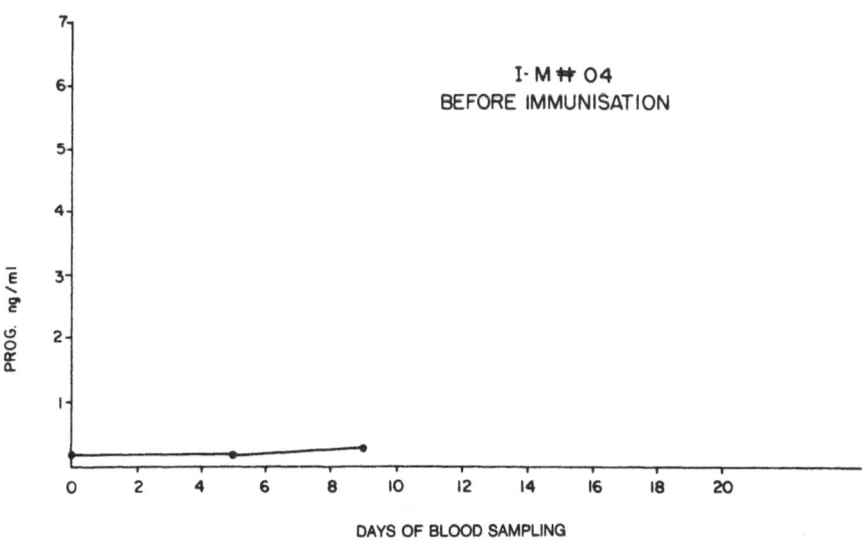

Figure 2 Progesterone levels in the peripheral plasma of non-immunized non-ovulating marmoset monkeys

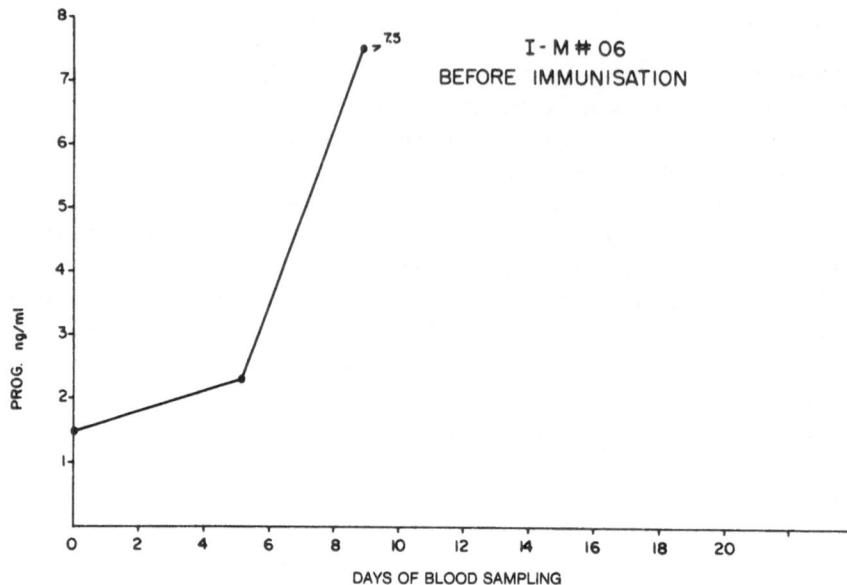

Figure 3 Progesterone levels in the peripheral plasma of non-immunized marmoset monkeys. Second control cycle

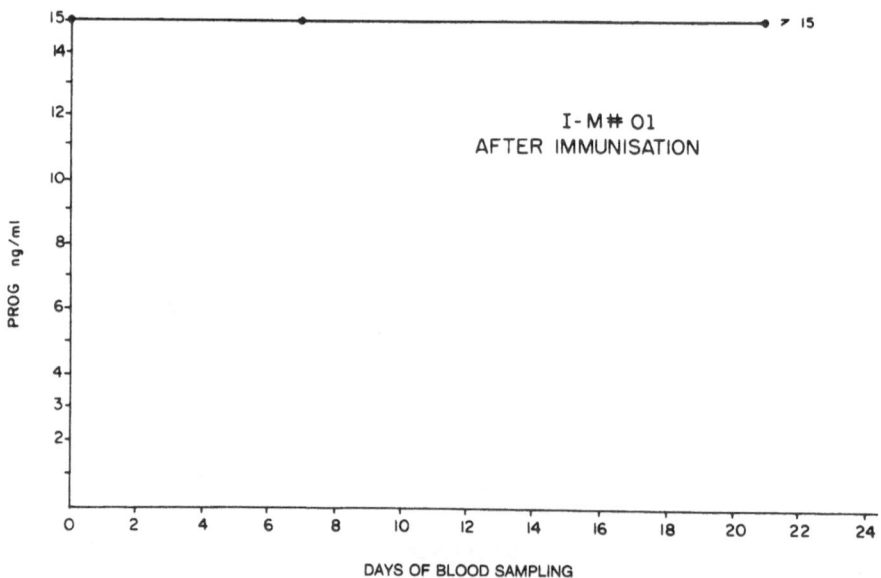

Figure 4 Progesterone levels in the peripheral plasma of immunized marmoset monkeys. These animals retained plasma progesterone levels above 15 μg/ml

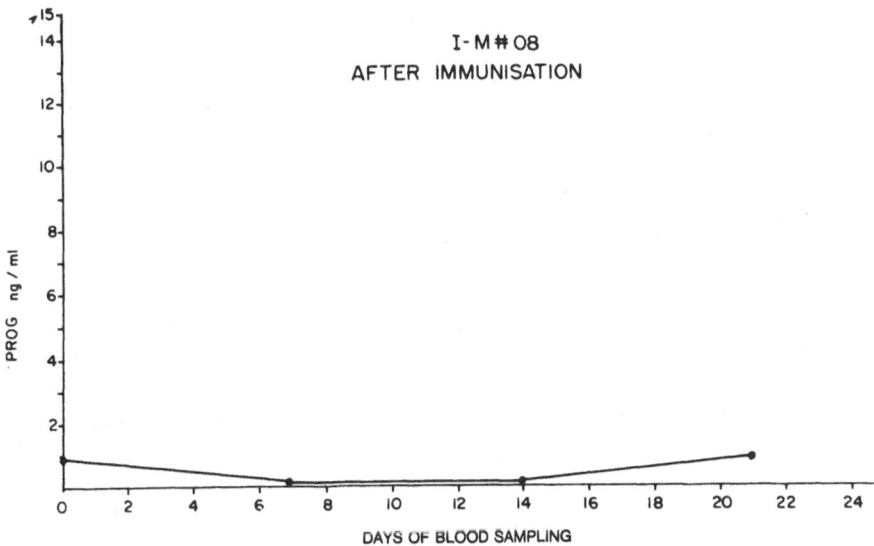

Figure 5 Progesterone levels in the peripheral plasma of immunized marmoset monkeys. In the other animals the plasma progesterone levels were below $3.0 \mu g/ml$

DISCUSSION

Thau reported that active immunization of female rhesus monkeys with oLH Beta caused a significant reduction in pregnancy rates, and that the contraceptive action could be reversed by administration of the progestin medroxy-progesterone acetate (MPA)[5]. Hearn immunized female marmosets actively and passively with the beta subunit of human chorionic gonadotrophin (hCG beta), reporting disruption of early pregnancy and that active immunization could also cause a marked reduction in the subsequent fertility of these animal[6]. We have previously reported that active immunization of female rhesus monkeys with oLH Beta caused multiple endocrinological effects on cycling and pregnant rhesus monkeys; such as impaired luteal function, the absence of 'corpus luteum rescue', decrease of progesterone and 17-OH-progesterone concentrations during the second and third trimester of gestation, and marked elevation in oestradiol concentrations of immunized animals throughout pregnancy[7].

Our study shows that active immunization against oLH Beta can impair normal corpus luteum function or disrupt early pregnancy.

The most likely explanation is that the antibodies to oLH Beta are blocking the luteotrophic stimulus from the embryo to the corpus luteum, and may even be acting on the pre-implantation blastocyst to prevent implantation. There was no interruption of the ovarian cycle after immunization against oLH Beta, indicating that a cross-reaction exists with the antibodies and the LH or FSH, but without preventing ovulation.

Improved methods of fertility regulation are essential. A promising approach to contraception is based on active immunization with pregnancy-specific antigen. An antigen which induces the production of circulating antibodies to chorionic gonadotrophin, neutralizing its biological activity, may form the basis of an antifertility vaccine.

SUMMARY

Marmoset monkeys (*Callithrix jacchus*) were actively immunized against chorionic gonadoptropin by injections of the beta fraction of ovine luteinizing hormone (oLH Beta). The immunizing emulsion was prepared by dissolving 50 μg, of oLH Beta in 250 μl, of saline emulsified with an equal volume of Freund's complete adjuvant. Multiple sites were injected subcutaneously in all animals on day 0 and 3 weeks later. Blood samples were drawn every week between 0900 and 1200 hours and plasma stored at −20 °C until assayed. Plasma levels of progesterone were determined by RIA in two complete cycles before immunization, and weekly thereafter. In three out of eight treated animals ovulation did not occur following immunization. In the other five animals ovulation occurred, indicating that no cross-reactivity with LH occurred.

ACKNOWLEDGEMENTS

This work was supported by the Rockefeller Foundation. The oLH Beta was kindly supplied by Dr M. R. Sairam, Director, Reproduction Research Laboratory, Montreal, Canada.

References

1. Stevens, V. C. (1974). Fertility control through active immunization using placenta proteins. In Diczfalusy, E. (ed.) *Immunological Approaches to Fertility Control*. pp. 357–69, Karol Symp. 7
2. Hearn, J. P. (1976). Immunization against pregnancy. *Proc. R. Soc. Lond. B.*, **195**, 149–60
3. Talwar, G. P., Sharma, N. C., Dubey, S. K., Salanhuddin, M., Das, C., Ramakrishnam, S., Kumar, S. and Hingorani, V. (1976). Immunization against human chorionic gonadotropin with conjugates of processed B-subunit of the hormone and tetanus toxoid. *Proc. Natl. Acad. Sci.*, **73**, 218–22
4. Sundaram, K., Chang, C. C., Laurence, K. A., Brinson, A. O., Atkinson, L. E., Segal, S. J. and Ward, D. N. (1976). The effectiveness in rhesus monkeys of an antifertility vaccine based on neutralization of chorionic gonadotropin. *Contraception*, **14**, 639–53
5. Thau, R. B. and Sundaram, K. (1980). The mechanism of action of an antifertility vaccine in the Rhesus monkey: reversal of the effects of antisera to the B-subunit of ovine luteinizing hormone by medroxyprogesterone acetate. *Fertil. Steril.*, **33**, 317–20
6. Hearn, J. P., Short, R. V. and Lunn, S. F. (1976). The effects of immunizing marmost monkeys against the B-subunit of hCG. In Edwards, R. G. and Johnson, M. H. (eds.) *Hormones*. pp. 229–47. (Cambridge University Press)

7. Spinola, P. G., Seidman, L. S., Sundaram, K. and Thau, R. B. (1982). Impaired steroid-ogenesis in the luteal phase of the reproductive cycle and during pregnancy in rhesus monkeys immunized with the B-subunit of ovine luteinizing hormone. *J.S. Biochem.*, 16, 151–6

Section 3

Vaginal and Intra-Uterine Contraception

19
Clinical and experimental evaluation of a new vaginal contraceptive

R. ERNY AND M. LEVRIER

INTRODUCTION

Benzalkonium chloride tampons represent an undeniable improvement in the local contraception field. They consist of a cylindrical polyvinyl alcohol sponge measuring 4 cm in diameter and 2.5 cm in length. This sponge is impregnated with 5 g of 1.2% benzalkonium chloride emulsion. Benzalkonium chloride is a strong spermicide included in the cationic detergent class, also called the 'saponiums'. It is a quaternary ammonium cationic surfactant which is not absorbed into the general circulatory system[1].

The effect of these new contraceptive sponges is immediate and lasts for 24 hours. Therefore, they have the advantage of being introduced several hours before sexual intercourse.

EFFICACY

Benzalkonium chloride tampons seem more effective than the other vaginal contraceptives. Serfaty[2] has tested the sponge in 118 fertile women for a total of 771 months. He observed two unexpected pregnancies, which occurred after misuse of the product. Cohen[3] has tested the sponge in 112 women for 1210 cycles. He observed one pregnancy in a patient who did not use the tampon for all sexual encounters.

Our study of 44 patients during 547 cycles gave one failure, this patient did not use the tampon.

Results

Efficacy of the tampons is very good, especially if used by selected women who are already users of a vaginal contraceptive method.

The failure rate was within 2–12% depending on the prescriber and the user of the vaginal contraception. Failures due to the product itself seem to be rare compared to those due to a misunderstanding or a misuse of the method. That is why the prescriber takes a prominent part by explaining the method in detail, and by selecting suitable patients. He must, therefore, exclude those women whom for different reasons such as understanding, motivation, sexuality or cultural context cannot conform to the requirements of the method or to its conditions of use.

EFFECTS OF THE TAMPON ON THE CERVICO-VAGINAL MUCOSA

We wanted to verify the negative effects resulting from a prolonged use of the tampon.

Twenty-seven women (20–45 years old) kept the tampon in the vagina for 24 hours. The cervical cytology was not modified. The colposcopic aspect remained the same. A vaginal biopsy was performed at the zone of support of the tampon, and the vaginal mucosa appeared normal.

EFFECTS OF THE TAMPON ON THE VAGINAL FLORA

We also wanted to verify if prolonged use of the tampon increased the risk of infections caused by an increase in the vaginal flora.

Our study was performed on 69 patients (20–45 years old) and affected by leukorrhoea. An ecouvillon sample was obtained. After gynaecological examination, a contraceptive sponge was introduced through the speculum by means of long forceps, in order to eliminate contamination by the perineal flora. Patients were asked to come back after 24 hours. Meanwhile they were asked not to wash the vagina and to abstain from any intercourse. A second sampling was done at withdrawal of the sponge. The study was completed by a bacteriological analysis of the withdrawn tampon in 26 patients.

Comments

Our bacteriological study is too limited, but confirms the results obtained in other studies. It dealt only with the more frequent vaginal organisms, and only gave an idea of the temporary effect of the local contraceptive.

The contraceptive sponge is active against Gram-positive cocci: streptococcus and staphylococcus, and Gram-negative cocci such as corynebacterium, enterobacters, *Escherichia coli*. Benzalkonium chloride is effective against trichomonas. We did not test the tampon against a cervico-vaginal gonococcus. But Siboulet and Catalan[4] have demonstrated the efficacy of benzalkonium chloride sponges against gonococcus. Therefore, the benzalkonium chloride sponge represents and interesting method of protection against sexually transmitted diseases.

The contraceptive sponge is very weakly active against lactobacillus, thus respecting the commensal flora and preserving the bacteriological equilibrium of the vagina. It is not active against *Candida albicans*. No aggravation of vaginal candidosis was observed. It seems, however, that the elimination of *Candida albicans*, from the flora against which the product is active, can be an aggravating factor. This theoretical risk disqualifies the contraceptive sponge as a regular method of contraception for women with recurrent mycosis.

EFFECTS OF BENZALKONIUM CHLORIDE ON CERVICAL MUCUS

Ovulatory cervical mucus changes on contact with benzalkonium chloride from clear and transparent to a coagulated thick mass forming a gelified magma at the cervical opening.

Using the technique of Chretien[5], this phenomenon was observed under the scanning electronic microscope. At low magnification, the reticulated cross-ruled screen is absent and a compact stiff mass is observed.

At medium magnification, the hazy and curdle aspects are more numerous. The thicker fibres are the only ones remaining, giving a hazy appearance at their intersections. The more impregnated samples with benzalkonium chloride give a compact aspect looking like a snow-covered landscape. However, the mucus is constantly flowing in the cervix which is, therefore, impregnated by a constantly renewed secretion. Benzalkonium chloride does not penetrate the cervix and does not form a stopper with local action.

CONCLUSION

Benzalkonium chloride is a spermicide which does not penetrate the general circulatory system. The tampon impregnated with benzalkonium chloride has a very good contraceptive efficacy lasting for 24 hours. The tampon is very well tolerated by the vaginal mucosa. The commensal vaginal flora is respected while numerous pathogenic organisms usually sexually transmitted are destroyed. This antiseptic property gives the sponge an important advantage in the prophylaxis of sexually transmitted diseases.

Unfortunately, candida is not influenced. Ovulatory cervical mucus rapidly changes to thick and coagulated on contact with benzalkonium chloride. But the importance of the effect on the cervical mucus on the contraceptive activity of benzalkonium chloride tampons remains mild.

113

References

1. Bleau, G. Non-absorption of benzalkonium chloride by the vaginal wall (to be submitted to) *J. Pharmacol. Sci.*
2. Serfaty, D. (1982). Le tampon contraceptif. *Entret. Bichat. Thérapeut.*, 225-8
3. Cohen, J. (1983). Expérimentation d'un tampon synthétique à usage uniqe imprégné de chlorure de benzalkoniu. *Contracep., Fertil., Sexual.*, 11, 131-3
4. Siboulet, A., Catalan, F., Bohbot, J. M. and Siboulet, A. (1982). Prévention des maladies sexuellement transmissibles. *Bull. Mém. Soc. Méd. Paris*, No. 4
5. Chretien, F. C. (1975). Préparation du mucus cervical à l'observation au microscope électronique à balayage. *J. Microsc. Biol. Cell.*, 24, 23-44

20
Benzalkonium chloride – a new vaginal contraceptive

B. N. BARWIN

MATERIALS AND METHODS

Pharmatex cones* have a cylindrical form with conical ends measuring 1.5 cm and weighing 1.6 g blended in a concentration 1.18% with a melting point lower than 37 °C. The shelf life at room temperature, has been established as better than 3 years. On melting, the suppository covers the mucous membrane of the vagina with a protective film, which because of its viscosity, reduces the

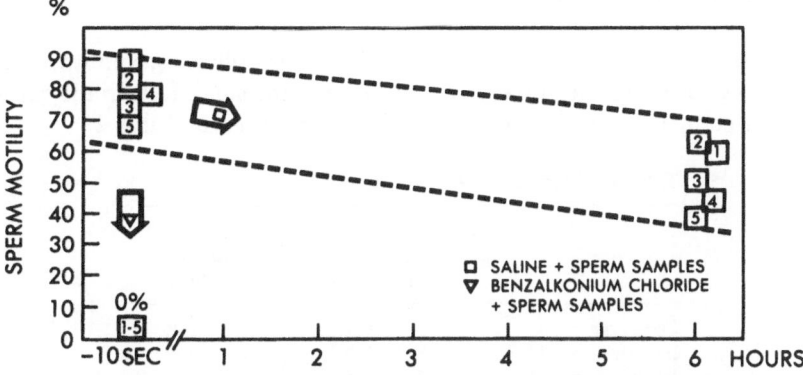

Figure 1 Observations of sperm motility. Fresh samples of donor sperm divided into 2 parts. Addition of benzalkonium chloride (diluted 1 part to 10 parts) resulted in prompt cessation of sperm motility within 10 seconds. ∇ normal saline dilution 1:10 was added to the second sample and sperm motility observed after 6 hours □

*Supplied by Interpharm, Laval, Quebec

115

migration of spermatozoa and combined with the wetting action of the benzalkonium chloride ensures a uniform and thorough covering; thus providing a dual physical and chemical action (Figure 1).

Eighty patients, aged 18–42 years, requesting vaginal contraception, were voluntarily enrolled for the study. Sixty patients were multiparae (10 postpartum) while 20 were nulliparous.

RESULTS

There were two pregnancies in this series both related to patient failure. The first patient did not re-insert a second Pharmatex Cone having had coitus the night before when she had used the vaginal cone. The second patient thought she was menstruating and did not utilize the cone. On further study of the menstrual calendar, she in fact had midcycle bleeding (Table 1).

Table 1   Pharmatex – pregnancy rates

	No. of patients	No. of cycles	No. of pregnancies	Pearl index
Crimail[1]	81	1228	5*	0.97
Bonhomme[2]	159	1492	1*	0.8
Levrier[3]	350	7140	4*	0.6
Leroy and Serror[4]	506	1470	2*	1.63
Gazave and Chatain[5]	144	3393	4*	1.41
Barwin[6]	80	1220	2*	0.8
Total	1320	15 943	16	1.33

*Uncorrected due to patient failure

Two patients complained of mild penile discomfort following coitus. Cultures for these couples were negative. A comparison of the side effects in the current literature compared with the present study is presented in Table 2.

Table 2   Pharmatex – side effects

	No. of patients (%)			
	Literature (487)		Barwin (80)	
Discharge	2	0.4	1	1.25
Irritation	5	1.0	0	0
Warm sensation	2	0.4	2	2.5
Burning	9	1.8	2	2.5
Male discomfort	4	0.8	1	1.25
Total	22	4.5	6	7.5

Reference 1, 7

The results of the Pap tests of the cervix at the commencement and conclusion of the study remained in the same class for all patients in the study.

The bactericidal properties of the ovule are shown in Figure 2 where patients were cultured prior to the commencement of the study and at one month. Bactericidal action is brought about by the elective destruction of the membrane of the micro-organism by the tensio-active properties of benzalkonium chloride[8].

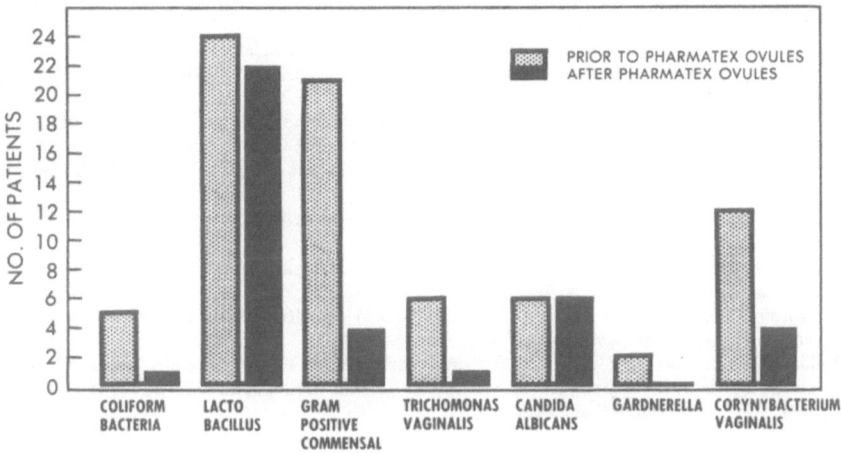

Figure 2 Comparison of bacterial cultures prior to and after the pharmatex ovules. Coliform bacteria include *Escherichia coli; Proteus mirabilis*. Gram-positive commensals include *Staphylococcus epidermis*, α-haemolytic streptococcus dipheroids

CONCLUSION

A clinical study in 80 women utilizing Pharmatex Cones (intravaginal chemical contraception) demonstrates good acceptability and tolerance with minimal side effects. The efficacy of this method in a well motivated, compliant patient is very acceptable. This method of contraception is ideal as an alternative where both the pill and the IUD are contra-indicated[9,10]. The longer duration of use (up to 4 hours) reduces the previous complaint of pre-coital interference [7-10].

Despite vaginal contraception being regarded as old-fashioned, unattractive, and relatively ineffective, it is now increasing in popularity[11-13]. Innovative studies in vaginal contraception with newer compounds such as benzalkonium chloride, with their greater effectiveness and acceptability, will allow vaginal contraception to take its proper place in the total contraceptive armamenterium.

References

1. Crimail, Ph. (1978). Indications, limites et résultats de la contraception intravaginale. *J. Agrégés*, **11**, 64–68
2. Bonhomme, J. – La contraception chimique locale. Résultats après quatre ans d'expérimentation. Sem. Hôp. Paris Thérapeutique, 1976, **52**, pp. 553–5; Entretiens de Bichat 1976, Thérapeutique, 189–91. Paris, Expansion scientifique française, 1977.
3. Levrier, M. (1978). La méthode chimique locale comme troisième voie en contraception. *Méd. Interne*, **13**, 663–5
4. Leroy, B. and Serror, R. (1979). Place d'une contraception par spermicide intravaginal dans le post-partum. *Rev. Fr. Gynecol.*, **74**, 63–5
5. Gazave, J. M. and Chatain, D. (1976). Plaidoyer pour la contraception locale. *Sud-Ou. Méd.*, **1**, No. 2
6. Barwin, B. N. (1983). Encare oval. A clinical study. *Contracept. Deliv. Syst.*, **4**, 331–4
7. Keith, L., Berger, G. S. and Jackson (1981). La contraception vaginale. *Contracept., Fertil., Sexual.*, **9**, 253–60
8. Dawson, R. (1966). The metabolism of animal phospholipids and their turnover in cell membranes. In *Essays in Biochemistry*. pp. 69. (Oxford: Oxford University Press)
9. Serfaty, D. (1978). La contraception mécanique: méthodes et indications. *Gaz. Méd. Fr.*, **85**, 3107–14
10. Serfaty, D. (1980). La contraception vaginale: réalité et perspectives. *Gaz. Méd. Fr.*, **87**, 29–34
11. Bonhomme, J. (1974). Efficacité et innocuité de la contraception par un spermicide intravaginal. *Med. Hosp.*, **10**, 419–22
12. Duthion, P. and Sénèze, J. (1979). Actualisation des données de la contraception intravaginale. *Actualités Gynecol.*, 10ᵉ Sér., 146–8
13. Duthion, P. and Sénèze, J. (1978). Etude et résultats en consultation hospitalière d'un contraceptif intravaginal. In *Entretiens de Bichat Thérapeutique*. pp. 141–2. (Paris: Expansion scientifique Française)

21
Contraception at caesarean delivery

M. N. PARIKH

INTRODUCTION

Proper spacing of pregnancies and limiting their number is very important not only for national programmes of population control but also for the health of the mother. A woman is most receptive to contraceptive advice at the time of her delivery or while undergoing induced abortion.

Postpartum contraception becomes vitally important when the woman is being delivered abdominally. A conception that quickly follows a caesarean section is taxing not only to the mother's well being but also to the uterine scar. Naturally, when a pregnancy occurs soon after a casearean delivery, the patient yearns for termination of such an unwanted and undesirable pregnancy. Terminating a pregnancy occurring in a recently scarred uterus is hazardous. All efforts must, therefore, be made to prevent an unwanted conception occurring in the post-caesarean period.

An intrauterine contraceptive device has great merits as a temporary contraceptive – the most important one being that it does not depend on the day-to-day motivation and co-operation of the patient. An IUCD inserted in the uterus prior to completion of involution carries a high risk of expulsion. Special long inserters have been devised to place the IUCD at the uterine fundus, during the immediate or early postpartum period, in an effort to reduce expulsion. Catgut sutures fixed to the upper limb of Lippes loop is yet another approach to the same problem.

It would be ideal to insert the IUCD after the involution is completed, but the majority of patients, especially in public hospitals in developing countries, do not come back even for routine post-partum examination. It is, therefore, necessary to find the ways and means of reducing the expulsion rate following immediate post-partum insertion of IUCD.

We believe that while performing a caesarean section an IUCD should be fixed to the fundus of the uterine cavity by catgut suture. By the time the catgut suture is absorbed the uterus is well on its way to involution, minimizing the chances of expulsion of IUCD. We wish to present here our preliminary experience in achieving reversible contraception at caesarean section using an IUCD in this fashion.

MATERIALS AND METHODS

While performing caesarean sections in 50 patients Multiload Cu 250 was fixed in the uterine cavity. Twenty patients were primigravidae. Fourteen patients were undergoing their second caesarean delivery and two patients their third (Table 1). Most of the caesarean sections were emergency ones, only 11 being elective.

Table 1   Patient profile

Primigravidae	20 (40%)
Previous 1 C.S.	14 (28%)
Previous 2 C.S.	2 (4%)
Elective C.S.	11 (22%)
Emergency C.S.	39 (78%)
Living children at C.S.	
Nil	30 (60%)
One	19 (38%)
Two	1 (2%)

Thirty patients had no living child at the time of this caesarean delivery, while 19 had one living child and 1 had two living children. Used in this way Multiload Cu 250 formed an effective method of birth spacing following caesarean section. Incidentally, only 10 patients were more than 25 years of age.

After delivering the fetus and removing the placenta the uterus is delivered out from the abdomen through the laparotomy wound. In our experience this can be done easily even through a low Pfannenstiel incision.

A '0' chromic catgut strand is tied at the junction of the vertical and the curved limbs of the Multiload Cu 250 by a single knot, leaving both the ends of the catgut long, one end of which is held with artery forceps and the other end is threaded into a long straight round body needle. The straight round body needle is employed to take one end of this catgut through the wall of the uterine fundus at its centre, first from inside out (Figure 1) and then from outside in (Figure 2) at a distance of 5 mm. The two ends of the catgut are now tied inside the uterine cavity so as to anchor the IUCD at the fundus of the cavity (Figure 3). The threads of the IUCD are now pushed through the cervix into the vagina.

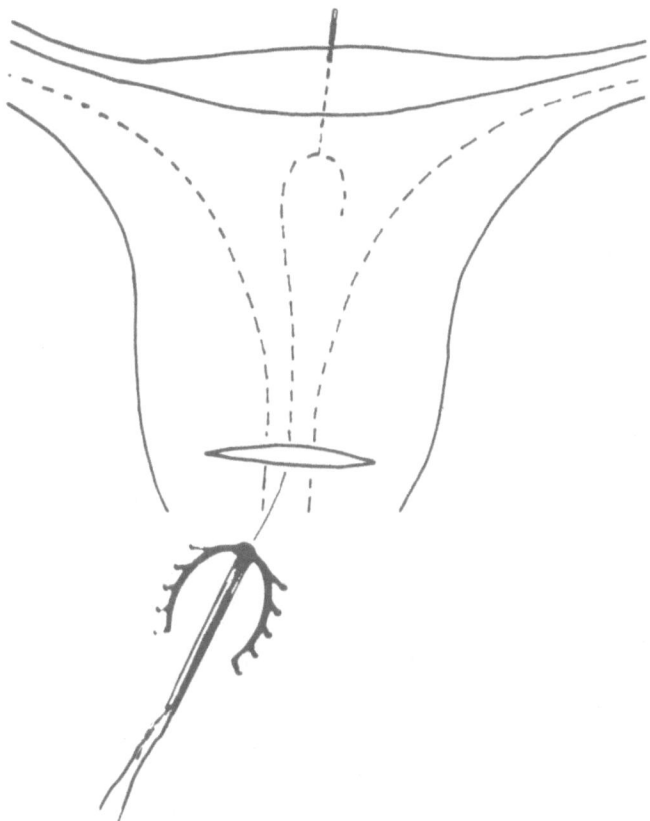

Figure 1

If the special Multiload Cu 250 with long threads meant for post-partum use is not available the threads of the ordinary Multiload Cu 250 can be lengthened by tying nylon strands to them.

The black thread of the IUCD is now anchored to the posterior wall of the uterus with '0' chromic catgut suture to prevent the somersaulting of the IUCD during the process of involution. The uterine incision and the abdomen are now closed.

On the 8th post-operative day a *per speculum* examination is done and the tail of the IUCD is cut just 1 cm beyond the external os of the cervix (Table 2).

RESULTS

At the 8th day examination the IUCD was found expelled in the vagina in one case. For some inexplicable reason the catgut stitch anchoring the IUCD to the

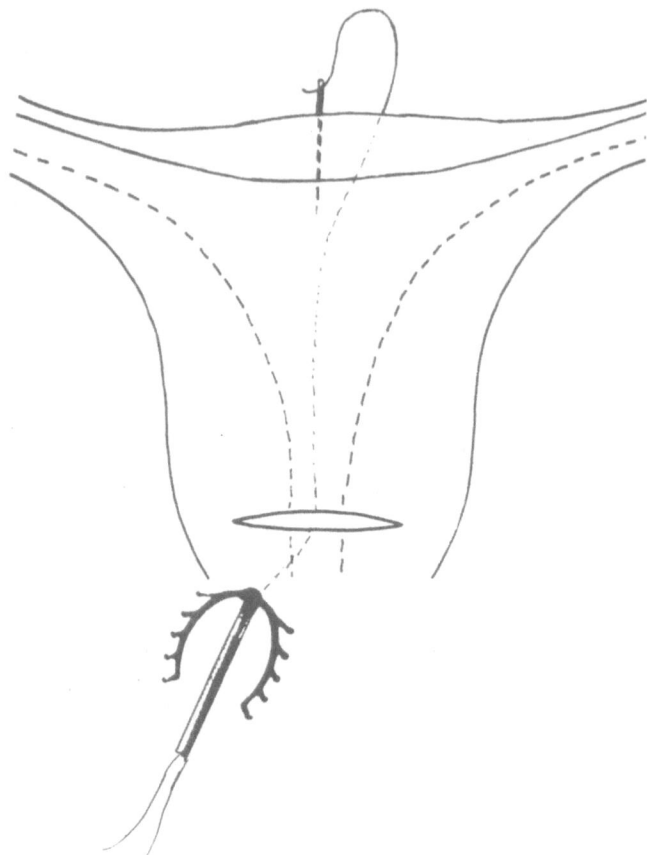

Figure 2

uterus might have been absorbed too soon, or perhaps the IUCD was not properly anchored to the uterus due to faulty technique. This was our 11th case.

The patient is again examined at the end of 6 weeks after delivery (Table 3). At this moment, four patients are not yet 6 weeks post-partum. The threads of the IUCD could be seen on speculum examination in 38 cases. One patient was lost to follow up.

In one case the IUCD was found expelled on the 8th day, as mentioned above. In one case IUCD was found expelled on the 13th post-operative day. This patient was in labour for more than 20 hours, had many vaginal examinations, was potentially infected at the time of caesarean section and developed puerperal sepsis. At present we avoid fixing IUCD at caesarean section in such potentially infected cases. In the remaining five cases although the threads of

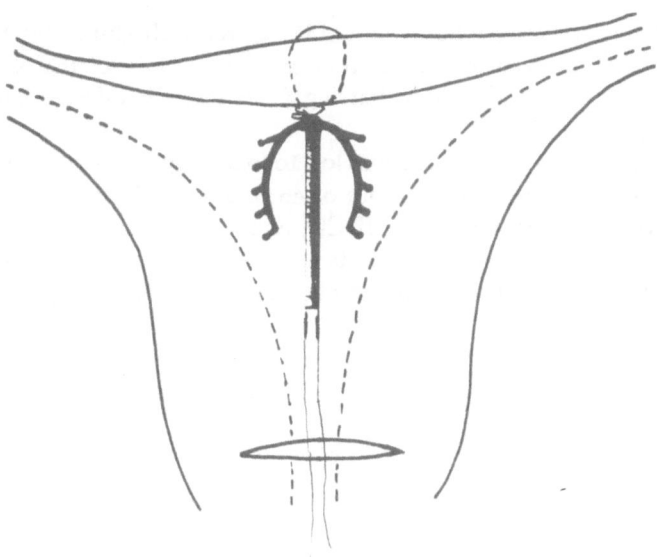

Figure 3

Table 2 8 days post-partum

IUCD expelled	1 ⎤
IUCD threads seen	46 ⎬ 50
IUCD threads not seen	3 ⎦

IUCD in uterus on ultrasound	Lost to follow up
2	1

Table 3 6 weeks post-partum

IUCD expelled	2 ⎤ 3/46 (6.5%)
Lost to follow up	1 ⎦
IUCD threads seen	38
IUCD threads not seen	5 (IUCD in uterus)
Total	46

the IUCD could not be seen ultrasound examination confirmed that the IUCD was in the uterine cavity. All these five cases are from amongst our first 20 cases. In two of these five cases the IUCD had somersaulted or turned upside down. In our effort to prevent such an occurrence we now anchor the threads of the IUCD to the posterior uterine wall. I would like to emphasize that in each

123

one of our last 30 cases, who have had the 6 weeks check-up, the threads of the IUCD could be seen on speculum examination. None of the patients had any side effects or complications, barring the potentially infected patient who developed puerperal sepsis.

Presuming that the patient who was lost to follow-up had expelled her IUCD, the expulsion rate works out at 3 out of 46 or 6.5%. This is remarkably low for a post-placental introduction of IUCD, and we feel that with experience the actual expulsion rate may turn out to be even lower. In our experience this approach to contraception at caesarean delivery is very rewarding indeed.

22
The combined Multiload Copper 250-Short IUD in women with reduced uterine cavity measurements

N. D. GOLDSTUCK

INTRODUCTION

Clinical uterine metrology was first attempted in 1894 by Haviland, using calipers, but it is only recently that clinical uterine metrology has come to play a role in IUD selection and design. Present day IUDs have been designed on the basis of uterine cavity measurements obtained from morbid anatomical and pathological studies, as well as from hysterography and ultrasound data[1]. These results are subject to error and it is only clinical uterine metrology which can determine uterine cavity size *in vivo*.

Thus, modern day IUDs are not compatible with the size of the uterine cavity into which they are to be inserted. This paper examines the performance of the Multiload Copper 250-Short (ML Cu 250 Short) IUD in a group of nulliparous women with short uterine cavity length, and examines the relationship of IUD size to IUD performance.

IUD PERFORMANCE AND UTERINE SIZE

Gibor *et al.*[2] showed that event rates following the insertion of the Cu 7 device were related to the total uterine length. Later Hasson *et al.*[3] showed that the critical factor in IUD performance was not the overall uterine length, but the length of the uterine cavity. Best IUD results (lowest event rates) were obtained when the uterine cavity was between 1.25 and 1.75 cm larger than the IUD which was inserted. Uterine cavity length measurements were made with Wing

Sound I which cannot measure uterine cavity width, and so Hasson did not consider the relationship of IUD width to uterine cavity width.

COMBINED MULTILOAD Cu 250-SHORT IN NULLIPAROUS WOMEN WITH SHORT UTERINE CAVITY LENGTH

Following a relatively unsuccessful trial with the Multiload Copper 250 mini in nulliparous women having short uterine cavities, it was decided to conduct a similar study with the Multiload Copper 250-Short IUD in a similar group of patients. A more successful outcome was confidently predicted because it was felt that the lateral dimensions of the ML Cu 250 'mini' were too narrow compared to the ML Cu 250 'short' (Table 1). This assumption was made following

Table 1   Dimensions of Multiload Cu 250 IUDs

	Vertical (mm)	Horizontal* (mm)	$\frac{Horizontal}{Vertical}$ (R)
ML Cu 250	36	18 (9)	0.5
ML Cu 250-short	25	18 (9)	0.72
ML Cu 250-mini	25	12 (7)	0.48

*Maximum width diameter. Figure in brackets is the distance in mm from the fundal tip of the device at which the maximum width diameter is obtained

a rigorous analysis of the relationship of IUD dimensions to event rates[4] including those of the 'mini' study. From the analysis an overall ratio (R) value for a number of IUDs was obtained. An overall ratio value for the uterine cavity of the nulliparous and multiparous uterus was also obtained (Figure 1). The results of these analyses suggested that the uterine cavity in the nulliparous woman was too wide for the ML Cu 250 'mini' but not for the ML Cu 250 'short'. The nulliparous uterine cavity appears to be functionally about 16 mm wide at a point about 1 cm below the fundus. This means that the flexible head of the fundally placed Multiload Copper 250 short will fit snugly into the nulliparous uterine cavity as the ML Cu 250 short is 18 mm wide at a point 1 cm below the fundal tip.

CLINICAL EXPERIENCE WITH THE MULTILOAD COPPER 250-SHORT IUD

Most standard copper bearing IUDs are 32–36 mm in length. Since many nulliparous women have uterine cavities which are shorter than this, they are often intolerent of standard copper bearing IUDs which impinge on the isthmus of the cervical canal.

Thirty women with uterine cavity length of less than 3.5 cm as determined with the Wing Sound I were selected for insertion of a ML Cu 250-short. Twenty of these women had used at least one or more standard copper bearing IUD.

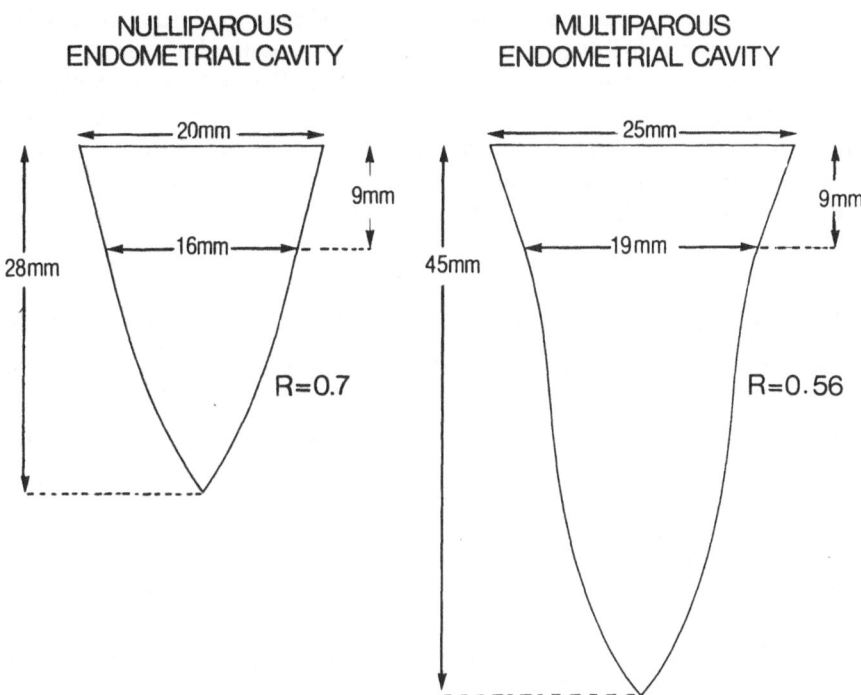

NULLIPAROUS
ENDOMETRIAL CAVITY

MULTIPAROUS
ENDOMETRIAL CAVITY

Figure 1 Dimensions and R values of nulliparous and multiparous endometrial cavities

All the patients who had used an IUD previously were forced to discontinue their use because of pain and/or bleeding, presumably because the standard size IUD encroached onto the cervical canal and isthmus leading to dysfunctional uterine contractions. At the end of a 6 month follow up period, two patients discontinued using the device, one because of persistent bleeding and a second expelled two ML Cu 250 short IUDs from a highly infantile type of uterus[5]. The subjects have now been followed up for nearly 3 years. There have been no further problems, and six devices have been removed so that the patients could have a planned pregnancy. The ML Cu 250 short IUD thus appears to be well suited to the nulliparous and small uterine cavity. In a larger study of the ML Cu 250 'short' on 813 women of whom 730 were nulliparous, with total uterine length of 5–7 cm, a 3 year cumulative expulsion rate of 4.9 and removal rate for bleeding and pain of 8.7 per 100 users was obtained[6].

DISCUSSION

Hasson has shown that uterine cavity length in nulliparous women is about 28–32 mm while Kurz[7] and Reynoso[8], using uterine calipers have shown that the uterine cavity width in nulliparae is of the order of 20–25 mm. Furthermore examination of IUD event rates in nulliparae in relation to dimensions of IUDs which are successful in this group suggests that devices with a horizontal : vertical ratio of around 0.7 are most suitable[4]. The ideal IUD for use in nulliparae should, therefore, (a) have a maximal width of less than 20 mm, (b) have a maximal length of less than 28 mm and (c) have an overall horizontal : vertical ratio of around 0.7 so as to fit into the dimensions of the uterine cavity as illustrated in Figure 1. The ML Cu 250 short fulfils all these requirements.

References

1. Hasson, H. M. and Dershin, H. (1981). Assessment of uterine shape by geometric means. *Contracept. Deliv. Syst.*, **2**, 59–76
2. Gibor, Y., Deysach, L. and Nissen, C. H. (1973). Uterine length: a prognostic indicator for the successful use of the Copper 7 intrauterine device. *J. Reprod. Med.*, **11**, 205–8
3. Hasson, H. M., Berger, G. S. and Edelman, D. A. (1976). Factors affecting intrauterine contraceptive device performance I. Endometrial cavity length. *Am. J. Obstet. Gynecol.*, **126**, 973–81
4. Goldstuck, N. D. (1982). The relationship of IUD dimensions to event rates. *Contracept. Deliv. Syst.*, **3**, 103–5
5. Goldstuck, N. D. (1981). A Critical ('Stress') evaluation of the Combined ML Cu 250-short IUD in nulliparous women. *Contracept. Deliv. Syst.*, **2**, 287–93
6. Van Os, W. A. A., Thiery, M., van der Pas, H., Rhemrev, P. E. R., de Nooyer, C. C. A. and Kleinhaut, J. (1981). Comparison of four different models of the Multiload Copper IUD. *Contracept. Deliv. Syst.*, **2**, 275–80
7. Kurz, K. H. (1981). Avoidance of the dimensional incompatibility as the main reason for side-effects in intrauterine contraception. *Contracept. Deliv. Syst.*, **2**, 21–9
8. Reynoso, L., Zamora, G., Gonzalez, M., Lozano, M. and Aznar, R. (1982). Uterine cavity measurement in Mexican women performed with the Batelle wing sound. *Contracept. Deliv. Syst.*, **3**, Abstr 182

23
Observations on the ML Cu 375

H. VAN DER PAS, M. THIERY AND W. VAN OS

INTRODUCTION

Gräfenberg, in 1929, first introduced the idea of inserting a large foreign object in the *cavum uteri* as a contraceptive device. For medical as well as political reasons, this method was discredited. It was not until the end of the 1950s that a new trial to insert inert material into the uterine cavity was made by some young research-workers[2].

Although nothing had been proved regarding the action of these IUDs, there was clear statistical evidence showing that the number of pregnancies could be significantly reduced in a normal fertile population and without serious medical side-effects. The following conclusion was made very soon: the greater the surface area of the foreign object, the lower the number of unwanted pregnancies. But unfortunately the medical side-effects increased with the growing surface area of the device. Things changed when Zipper[3] reduced surface area of the device and added copper to the inert model, resulting in a lower number of accidental pregnancies. It was Tatum[4] who later proved that the antifertility effect of the IUD was greater as the copper surface inserted in the *cavum uteri* was increased. But an unlimited addition of copper seemed inappropriate to him, so he limited the copper surface to $220 \, mm^2$.

Still later van Os[5] changed the original T-model and increased the surface copper into the uterine cavity to first $250 \, mm^2$, then $375 \, mm^2$.

Tietze and Lewit[6] defined a past life table method to investigate the effectiveness and acceptability of an IUD.

Our analysis of the ML Cu 375 fitted in 1969 patients over a period of 5 years or a total of 71 818 woman months of use (Table 1) indicated a very low rate of accidental pregnancies: 0.4, 1.6, 2.1, 2.8 and 3.2 after respectively 1, 2, 3, 4

129

Table 1 ML Cu 375

Events	12 m	24 m	36 m	48 m	60 m
Accidental pregnancy	0.4 (0.2–0.8)	1.6 (1.0–2.3)	2.1 (1.4–2.9)	2.8 (1.9–3.6)	3.2 (2.9–4.2)
Expulsion	1.8 (1.2–2.4)	2.3 (1.6–3.0)	2.7 (1.9–3.5)	3.6 (2.7–4.6)	4.0 (3.0–5.1)
Removals:					
bleeding/pain	5.9 (4.8–7.0)	10.8 (9.3–12.3)	14.7 (12.9–16.5)	18.5 (16.6–20.5)	21.2 (19.1–23.4)
other medical reasons	0.9 (0.4–1.3)	2.3 (1.5–3.0)	3.2 (2.3–4.1)	4.1 (3.0–5.2)	5.3 (4.0–6.6)
planned pregnancy	5.2 (4.2–6.3)	11.6 (10.0–13.1)	16.0 (14.2–17.9)	19.3 (17.3–21.4)	22.0 (19.8–24.1)
personal reasons	2.7 (1.9–3.4)	5.8 (4.7–7.0)	10.2 (8.6–11.7)	14.0 (12.1–15.8)	18.4 (16.2–20.6)
Continuation rate	85.0	70.3	59.5	51.3	44.3
investigator's choice	0.0 (0.0–0.2)	0.2 (0.0–0.6)	0.7 (0.3–1.3)	2.4 (1.4–3.3)	25.5 (21.7–29.2)
LFU	1.8 (1.2–2.4)	4.5 (3.4–5.5)	7.1 (5.7–8.5)	9.8 (8.2–11.5)	12.8 (10.8–14.7)
RFU	1.0 (0.6–1.5)	1.1 (0.6–1.6)	2.5 (1.6–3.3)	3.6 (2.6–4.6)	4.9 (3.6–6.2)
Woman-months of use	21 762	39 223	53 173	64 567	71 818

and 5 years. The IUDs had been inserted intermenstrually as well as postpartum and postabortum.

From our experience over the last years with this computer program we hope to prove that by increasing the amount of copper from 25 mm^2 to 375 mm^2 the rates of accidental pregnancies decrease, while the expulsion rates remain unchanged.

MATERIALS AND METHODS

The devices studied are the ML Cu 250 and ML Cu 375. The latter has the same skeleton as the standard (ML Cu 250) model, except for the larger copper surface area. Both models were inserted at interim (i.e. in non-gravid women, not earlier than 6 weeks after delivery or abortion) by the same team of gynaecologists using the standard technique, i.e. after sounding of the uterus, the device was inserted while keeping the uterine axis straight by means of a valsellum. The subjects were women requesting intrauterine contraception and having no contra-indications for use of the method, e.g. pelvic inflammatory disease (PID) or incipient pregnancy.

The subjects did not use any additional contraceptive method while under observation.

The difference between unwanted pregnancy rates in various studies of our group emanates from the fact that several investigators take part in multicentre publications and equally that the lost to follow-up (LFU) rates of the various studies are very different[7-9]. In a straight study of 877 patients (Table 2) fitted only at interim with a ML Cu 250 we noted respectively for 12 and 24 months an accidental pregnancy rate of 1.2 and 2.0 and an expulsion rate of 1.3 and 2.1 over the same period of time.

Comparing this study to another straight study by the same investigators, but exactly 2 years later – 1650 subjects at interim fitted with a ML Cu 375 (Table 3) which was new to the market, excluding the possibility of a randomized study – we found at 1 and 2 years a pregnancy rate of 0.3 and 1.5 and an expulsion rate of 1.5 and 2.0.

The difference between the accidental pregnancy rates in both series is clear. Moreover, pregnancies appear later with the ML Cu 375 than with the ML Cu 250. Also apparent is the fact that the rate of accidental pregnancies is equal 1 year after insertion of the ML Cu 250 and 2 years after insertion of the ML Cu 375. In order to make a precise analysis of these observations, and for better comparison of both groups a matched study was started.

Two groups of patients were compared. Members of the first (control) group were taken from a series of 1152 women using a ML Cu 250. Each member of the test group was matched with a woman belonging to the control group and three variables were used. First the ML Cu 375 devices were to be inserted in the same month as the corresponding ML Cu 350; however, because the clinical

Table 2   ML Cu 250 (No. of insertions: 877)

Events	12 m	24 m
Accidental pregnancy	1.2 (0.5–2.2)	2.0 (1.0–3.1)
Expulsion	1.3 (0.6–2.4)	2.1 (1.0–3.1)
Removals:		
bleeding/pain	5.7 (4.1–7.4)	10.7 (8.5–13.0)
other medical reasons	3.4 (2.1–4.6)	3.8 (2.5–5.2)
planned pregnancy	3.0 (1.8–4.3)	8.5 (6.4–10.7)
personal reasons	4.8 (3.3–6.3)	10.9 (8.6–13.2)
Continuation rate	82.7	32.3
investigator's choice	0.1 (0.0–0.6)	1.5 (0.7–2.8)
LFU	2.0 (1.0–3.0)	9.9 (7.5–12.2)
RFU	1.6 (0.7–2.5)	2.6 (1.4–3.8)
Woman-months of use	9440	16 761

Table 3   ML Cu 375 (No. of insertions: 1650)

Events	12 m	24 m
Accidental pregnancy	0.3 (0.1–0.8)	1.5 (0.2–2.1)
Expulsion	1.5 (0.9–2.1)	2.0 (1.6–2.7)
Removals:		
bleeding/pain	5.8 (4.6–7.0)	10.3 (8.7–11.9)
other medical reasons	1.0 (0.5–1.5)	2.4 (1.6–3.2)
planned pregnancy	4.7 (3.6–5.7)	10.0 (8.4–11.5)
personal reasons	2.7 (1.9–3.5)	6.1 (4.8–7.4)
Continuation rate	85.9	71.9
investigator's choice	0.0 (0.0–0.2)	0.2 (0.0–0.7)
LFU	1.0 (0.5–1.6)	3.0 (2.0–4.0)
RFU	1.0 (0.5–1.5)	1.1 (0.6–1.6)
Woman-months of use	18 333	33 322

trial of the ML Cu 375 started much later than of the standard model, there is a time difference of exactly 2 years between each ML Cu 375 subject and her matched control. Secondly, at the time of insertion matched pairs belonged to the same age group (i.e. either ≤30 years or >30 years of age) and were comparable for gravidity and parity.

The study was performed in a total of 912 women (Table 4) fitted with a ML copper device, 456 of them with the ML Cu 375 and 456 with the ML Cu 250. The present report concerns the observations made up to June 1, 1983 and covers a total of 25 180 woman months of use, 13 126 of them obtained with the experimental model (ML Cu 375).

The validity of the comparison of the two ML devices is enhanced by the fact that all cases were treated in the same clinic by the same investigators. Furthermore, the criteria applied to match propositae with controls included all major variables bearing on IUD performance. It should be added that cross-insertions of the two models did not occur, which implies that a ML Cu 375 model was

Table 4 Results of matched study (No. of insertions: 456 each device)

Events	ML Cu 375			ML Cu 250		
	12 m	24 m	36 m	12 m	24 m	36 m
Accidental pregnancy	0.2 (0.0–1.2)	0.8 (0.2–2.3)	1.5 (0.5–3.4)	2.2 (1.0–4.2)	3.1 (1.3–4.9)	3.8 (1.8–5.8)
Expulsion	0.5 (0.0–1.6)	1.0 (0.3–2.5)	1.7 (0.6–3.6)	0.7 (0.2–2.2)	1.0 (0.3–2.6)	1.4 (0.4–3.3)
Removals:						
bleeding/pain	4.1 (2.2–5.9)	10.5 (7.5–13.5)	13.5 (10.0–16.9)	5.6 (3.4–7.9)	9.5 (6.6–12.5)	10.8 (7.7–14.0)
other medical reasons	0.0 (0.0–0.8)	1.6 (0.6–3.4)	2.6 (1.9–4.9)	3.3 (1.6–5.1)	3.9 (2.0–5.8)	5.0 (2.7–7.2)
planned pregnancy	4.1 (2.2–6.0)	11.4 (8.3–14.6)	14.1 (10.6–17.6)	3.5 (1.6–5.3)	9.4 (6.4–12.4)	12.1 (8.6–15.6)
personal reasons	2.3 (1.1–4.3)	7.4 (4.8–10.1)	12.5 (9.0–15.9)	4.3 (2.3–6.2)	11.2 (8.0–14.4)	17.9 (13.8–21.9)
Continuation rate	90.4	72.1	61.3	83.1	68.2	58.5
investigator's choice	0.0 (0.0–0.8)	0.3 (0.0–1.7)	1.0 (0.2–2.9)	0.2 (0.0–1.3)	1.5 (0.5–3.4)	21.7 (16.6–26.7)
LFU	0.0 (0.0–0.8)	0.0 (0.0–0.8)	0.0 (0.0–0.8)	0.0 (0.0–0.9)	0.0 (0.0–0.9)	0.0 (0.0–0.9)
RFU	0.5 (0.1–1.7)	0.5 (0.1–1.7)	1.2 (0.3–3.0)	1.2 (0.4–2.71)	1.8 (0.7–3.7)	2.5 (1.2–4.8)
Woman-months of use	5245	9578	13126	4970	8919	12054

never inserted in a subject from whom a ML Cu 250 had been retrieved. The contraceptive effect of the ML Cu 375 is significantly greater ($p < 0.001$) than with the standard model. No perforations were diagnosed during the period covered by this report. This study confirms Tatum's original hypothesis, i.e. that the contraceptive effect increases in proportion to the surface area of copper[10]. Moreover, the increase in the surface area of copper to 375 mm^2 in the ML device corresponds to a statistically significant increase in its clinical efficacy. Finally, retention of the ML Cu 375 is similar to that of the standard model.

Attempting to explain the reason for these results we compared two other devices: the T Cu 200 and the T Cu 220 C[11] (Table 5). In a matched study over 1, 2 and 3 years, using the same criteria as mentioned above, accidental pregnancy rates for the T Cu 200 were 3.3, 3.3 and 4.0 but only 1.0, 2.6 and 3.2 for the T Cu 220 C. It appears to be the same trend as seen in observations made for the ML Cu 250 and the ML Cu 375, notwithstanding the small difference in surface area between the T Cu 200 and the T Cu 220 C of only 20 mm^2; this gives a 10% difference, whereas the difference between the ML Cu 250 and the ML Cu 375 is 50%.

The obvious question is whether the difference in surface area is the major factor in this case, for the copper is not only spread over the surface area but it has a volume too.

A third smaller study (Table 6) was made to compare copper volumes but it probably is not significant due to the small number of patients observed, however it does seem to support the hypothesis. We randomized three groups of patients fitted with T Cu 200, ML Cu 250 and ML Cu 375. The accidental pregnancy rates after 1, 2 and 3 years for the T Cu 200 are 3.4, 4.7 and 4.7 respectively; in the groups of patients fitted with ML Cu 250 and ML Cu 375 no pregnancies were observed. The results of the three studies have been summarized in a diagram (Figure 1) showing clear evidence of the superiority of the ML Cu 375. We presume that the great contraceptive difference in the first year of its use is due to the copper mass rather than to the surface of copper coils.

CONCLUSION

The results of these studies lead to some hypotheses which might explain the greater contraceptive effect of the ML Cu 375:

(1) The greater copper mass may, immediately after insertion, cause a greater leukotaxia which is permanent for some time.

(2) The greater copper mass can release more copper ions influencing the cervical mucus so that sperm penetration is decreased.

Table 5 Results of matched study (No. of insertions: 230 each device)

Events	T Cu 220C			T Cu 200		
	12 m	24 m	36 m	12 m	24 m	36 m
Accidental pregnancy	1.0 (0.1–3.5)	2.6 (0.8–6.0)	3.2 (1.2–6.9)	3.3 (1.3–6.9)	3.3 (1.3–6.9)	4.0 (1.8–7.9)
Expulsion	4.0 (1.8–7.5)	4.0 (1.8–7.5)	4.8 (2.2–8.4)	4.1 (1.9–7.8)	4.6 (2.2–8.5)	5.3 (2.2–8.3)
Removals:						
bleeding/pain	3.7 (1.6–7.2)	5.2 (2.2–8.3)	5.9 (2.6–9.2)	4.9 (2.4–9.0)	8.2 (4.3–12.1)	11.8 (7.1–16.6)
other medical reasons	1.0 (0.1–3.4)	1.5 (0.3–4.3)	1.5 (0.3–4.3)	1.5 (0.3–4.2)	1.5 (0.3–4.2)	1.5 (0.3–4.2)
planned pregnancy	3.3 (1.3–6.8)	9.4 (5.3–13.4)	12.7 (8.0–17.5)	2.9 (1.1–6.3)	6.2 (2.8–9.7)	8.1 (4.1–12.2)
personal reasons	0.0 (0.0–1.8)	2.7 (0.8–6.1)	4.5 (2.0–8.9)	1.5 (0.3–4.2)	3.7 (1.5–7.7)	5.6 (2.7–10.3)
Continuation rate	88.4	76.1	70.9	83.7	75.1	68.4
investigator's choice	0.0 (0.0–1.8)	0.0 (0.0–1.8)	0.6 (0.0–3.4)	1.0 (0.1–3.4)	1.0 (0.1–3.4)	14.5 (8.8–20.2)
LFU	1.4 (0.3–4.1)	5.4 (2.6–9.8)	8.5 (4.3–12.6)	3.0 (1.1–6.4)	3.5 (1.4–7.2)	7.9 (3.8–11.9)
RFU	0.5 (0.0–2.7)	1.0 (0.1–3.7)	2.3 (0.6–5.8)	0	0	0
Woman-months of use	2566	4768	6622	2451	4533	6336

Table 6 Comparison of ML Cu 375, ML Cu 250 and T Cu 200 (No. of insertions: 100 each device)

Events	ML Cu 375			ML Cu 250			T Cu 200		
	12 m	24 m	36 m	12 m	24 m	36 m	12 m	24 m	36 m
Accidental pregnancy	0.0	0.0	0.0	0.0	0.0	0.0	3.4 (0.7–9.9)	4.7 (1.3–12.0)	4.7 (1.3–12.0)
Expulsion	3.1 (0.7–9.1)	6.7 (2.5–14.4)	6.7 (2.5–14.4)	4.1 (1.1–10.4)	6.5 (2.4–14.0)	6.5 (2.4–0.0)	4.1 (1.1–10.4)	4.1 (1.1–10.4)	4.1 (1.1–10.4)
Removals:									
bleeding/pain	2.1 (0.3–7.6)	4.5 (1.2–11.9)	4.5 (1.2–11.9)	1.0 (0.03–5.8)	1.0 (0.03–5.8)	4.2 (0.9–00.0)	5.4 (1.7–12.6)	8.0 (3.2–16.4)	12.6 (6.1–23.1)
other medical reasons	1.0 (0.03–5.6)	2.3 (0.3–8.4)	2.3 (0.3–8.4)	0.0	0.0	0.0	0.0 (0.0–3.8)	1.2 (0.03–7.0)	1.2 (0.03–7.0)
planned pregnancy	3.3 (0.7–9.4)	8.0 (3.2–16.6)	12.3 (5.9–22.5)	2.1 (0.3–7.7)	6.8 (2.5–15.7)	9.6 (4.2–00.0)	2.2 (0.3–7.8)	9.9 (4.4–19.4)	12.7 (6.1–23.2)
personal reasons	0.0 (0.0–3.7)	0.0 (0.0–3.7)	1.4 (0.03–7.7)	0.0 (0.0–4.0)	2.4 (0.3–8.5)	5.4 (1.5–00.0)	1.2 (0.03–6.4)	3.8 (0.8–11.0)	3.8 (0.8–11.0)
Continuation rate	90.8	80.1	76.7	93.0	83.4	77.7	86.8	72.0	67.6
investigator's choice	0.0 (0.0–3.7)	1.3 (0.03–7.3)	23.3 (13.1–33.5)	2.2 (0.3–7.9)	3.4 (0.7–9.9)	23.3 (13.1–00.0)	0.0 (0.0–3.8)	0.0 (0.0–3.8)	15.3 (7.0–28.8)
LFU	5.3 (1.7–12.3)	6.6 (2.4–14.3)	10.7 (4.9–20.1)	3.1 (0.7–9.1)	6.8 (2.5–14.7)	15.0 (7.1–00.0)	3.4 (0.7–10.0)	6.2 (2.0–14.4)	10.7 (4.7–21.6)
RFU	1.2 (0.03–6.5)	1.2 (0.03–6.5)	1.2 (0.03–6.5)	0.0 (0.0–4.0)	2.5 (0.3–8.9)	3.9 (0.8–00.0)	0.0 (0.0–3.8)	1.3 (0.03–7.4)	1.3 (0.03–7.4)
Woman-months of use	1110	2040	2815	1131	2101	2887	1064	1948	2695

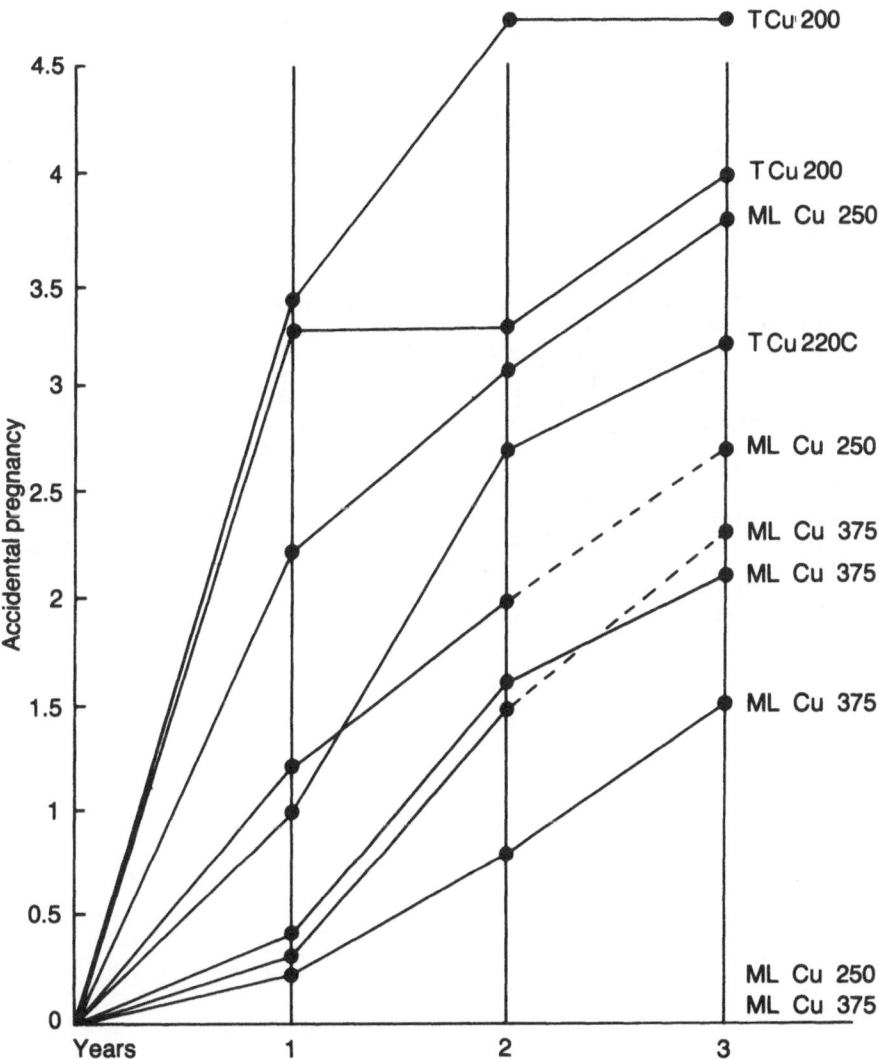

Figure 1

If our hypotheses are correct, they may add weight to the argument for insertion of IUDs with a greater copper content, and for a yearly change in the IUD, resulting in a negligible rate of unwanted pregnancies for high-risk patients.

137

References

1. Gräfenberg, E. (1929). Die intrauteriene Methode der Konzeption verhütung. In Trench, Trulmer, Haire, N. and Kegan, P. (eds.) *IIIe Congress of the World League for Sexual Reform*, London.
2. Lippes, J. A., Zielezny, M. (1975). The loop after two years. In Hefnani, F., Segal, S. J. (eds.) *Analysis of Intrauterine Contraception*. pp. 225–36. (Amsterdam: North Holland)
3. Zipper, J., Medel, M. and Prager, R. (1969). Suppression of fertility by intrauterine copper and zinc in rabbits: a new approach to intrauterine contraception. *Am. J. Obstet. Gynecol.*, 105, 529–34
4. Tatum, J. J. (1973). Metallic copper as an intrauterine contraceptive agent. *Am. J. Obstet. Gynecol.*, 117, 602–18
5. Van Os, W., Rhemrev, P. E., Bomert, L. and Aartsen, E. J. (1979). Experience with a combined multiload contraceptive intrauterine device. Presented at the *VIIIth World Congress on Fertility and Sterility*. Abstract 165. November 3–9, Buenos Aires
6. Tietze, C. and Lewit, S. (1970). Evaluation of intrauterine devices: ninth progress report of the cooperative statistical programme. *Stud. Fam. Plann.*, 55, 1–40
7. Thiery, M., Van der Pas, H., Delbeke, L. and Van Kets, H. (1980). Comparative performance of two copper-wired IUDs. *Contracept. Deliv. Syst.*, 1, 27–35
8. Van Kets, H., Thiery, M., Van der Pas, H. *et al.* (1980). Interim insertion of the ML Cu 250 intrauterine contraceptive device. *Contracept. Deliv. Syst.*, 2, 149–54
9. Thiery, M., Van der Pas, H., Van Os, W. *et al.* (1979). Three years experience with the ML Cu 250, a new copper-wired intrauterine contraceptive device. *Br. J. Fam. Plann.*, 5, 36–8
10. Tauber, P. F., Van der Pas, H., Thiery, M. and Ludwig, H. (1978). Copper as an antifertility agent in intrauterine devices. *IRCS Med. Sci.*, 6, 527
11. Van der Pas, H., Thiery, M., Delbeke, L., Van Kets, H. and Haspels, A. (1980). Six years experience with the T Cu 220 C intrauterine contraceptive device. *Contracept. Deliv. Syst.*, 1, 1–10

24
Copper medicated IUDs are not associated with abortion

K. H. KURZ, F. LEIDENBERGER AND P. MEIER-OEHLKE

To determine the rate of implantation, β-hCG was determined by radio-immunoassay in a total of 368 regularly cohabitating, highly fertile women (84% were aged 20–34) bearing symmetrical, copper-medicated IUDs (T Cu 200 adapted and Multiload Cu 250) or not using contraception.

They were divided into four groups (Table 1):

Group 1   In 109 IUD amenorrhoeic women, blood samples were taken after day 30 of that cycle. Where ultrasonography uncovered a gestation sac, these women were excluded. In two cases from Group 1, β-hCG was increased (>25 mIU), pregnancy was determined by ultrasonography later and continued. 107 women later menstruated primarily during the 2 weeks subsequent to the blood tests.

Group 2   In a control group of 177 non-contraceptive users β-hCG was elevated in 59 cases (33%) indicating the occurrence of implantation. In all cases, pregnancy was confirmed later by ultrasonography.

Group 3   Blood samples were taken during day 23–27 of the cycle in 28 IUD women with regular cycles. β-hCG was not elevated in any case.

Group 4   In the control group of 54 non-contraceptive users, increased β-hCG levels were found during day 23–27 of the cycle in 14 cases (26%). Most of these women asked for an early determination of pregnancy.

In 1979, Nilson and co-workers[1] published the finding of two positive β-hCG values out of 102 women using Cu IUDs. They also determined LH progesterone levels. Monitoring the two cases, β-hCG could not be detected 3 days later.

139

Table 1 Determination of β-hCG

Copper-IUD	Number of women (n = 368)	Taking out (day of cycle)	Pregnant (25 mIU positive)	Non-pregnant (25 mIU negative)
1. +	n = 109	30+	2 (1.8%)	107 (98.2%)
2. −	n = 177	30+	59 (33.3%)	118 (66.7%)
3. +	n = 28	23–27	0 (0%)	28 (100%)
4. −	n = 54	23–27	14 (25.9%)	40 (74.1%)

The investigators suggested that the β-hCG would have been produced by blastocysts not yet implanted.

In view of the statement that life as a human being begins with full implantation (a.o. Governmental law of the Federal Republic of Germany, declaration of the American Society of Gynaecology and Obstetrics, etc.) the above results prove that copper IUDs do not act as abortifacients. Further reports refer to the effective spermatotoxic mode of action of symmetrical copper IUDs. In contrast to plastic-only IUDs, an inhibition of sperm mobility and migration in the cervical mucus of copper IUD bearers by other workers[2–5]. The same goal was reached by copper ionization of the rabbit and human cervix[6] and of the ductus deferens of rats and rabbits.

No sperm could be found in the tubal fluid after cohabitation or artificial insemination during midcycle in ectomized oviducts of IUD bearers[8] (and Zipper, personal communication 1983). Plastic IUDs did not show inhibition of sperm ascension as was found in the groups with copper IUDs. No spermatozoa were found in the peritoneal fluid of women with the symmetrical copper IUD, Multiload Cu 250[9, 10].

EPF (early pregnancy factor) was positive in four out of eight cycles in four women bearing plastic IUDs (50%), and in two out of eight cycles of six women with the 7 Cu 200 devices (25%), EPF was *negative* in all four cycles of two women with T Cu 200 IUDs (100%)[11]. EPF is controversial among experts.

As so often happens in the biological sciences, there is a tendency to assume that the discovery of a physiological phenomenon in one animal can be universally applied[12]. The hypotheses that symmetrical IUDs medicated with sufficient amounts of high-quality copper (e.g. Multiload 250/375 and T Cu 200, 220, 380) mainly act toxically on the blastocyst as abortifacients, is based on results found in animals, particularly small laboratory animals such as rodents.

There are fundamental anatomical and physiological differences amongst mammalian species, e.g. form and size of the genital tract, the amount of ejaculate, the total number of spermatozoa, the efficiency of the cervical mucus barrier and the site of deposition of spermatozoa, e.g. uterine cavity, and suction effects with a positive influence on sperm transport being different from sperm migration.

SUMMARY

Symmetrical copper-bearing intrauterine devices which continuously release a sufficient number of copper ions have a spermatotoxic effect in humans, directly and/or indirectly via intermediary products of endometrial metabolism and uterine, tubal and cervical secretions. As a result, the estimated 40–50% natural early abortions occurring without the use of contraception, which are attributed to 'abundance of nature', could also be prevented. To correct nature has been a basic aim in medicine for thousands of years.

Should the leading consensus of opinion insist that copper-bearing intrauterine devices generally or predominantly act as nidation inhibitors, we feel that we can now justifiably demand conclusive evidence on this point in the light of recent findings.

References

1. Nilsson, C. G., Lähteenmäki, P. and Luukkainen, T. (1979). Detection of beta subunit HCG in plasma of IUD users as an indication of frequency of conception. *Int. J. Fertil.*, **24**, 134
2. Kesserü, E., Camacho-Ortega, P. (1972). Influence of metals on in vitro sperm migration in the human cervical mucus. *Contraception*, **6**, 231
3. Ullman, G., Hammerstein, J. (1972). Inhibition of sperm motility in vitro by copper wire. *Contraception*, **6**, 71
4. Hefnawi, F., Kandil, O., Askalani, A., Serour, I. (1975). Mode of action of the copper IUD: Effect on endometrial copper and cervical mucus sperm migration. In *Analysis of Intrauterine Contraception*, Hefnawi, F. and Segal, S. J., eds. pp. 459–63. (Amsterdam: North-Holland)
5. Ros, A., Piemonte, G., Rugiati, S. (1980). Copper IUD emission and its effects on human cervical mucus-spermatozoa interaction. *Contracept. Deliv. Syst.*, **1**, 113
6. Chattopadhyay, S. K., Ahuja, J. M. and Khanna, S. D. (1976). Effect of copper ionisation of the cervix on sperm migration. *Contraception*, **14**, 331
7. Riar, S. S., Sawney, R. C., Bardhan, J., Thomas, P., Jain, R. K. and Kain, A. K. (1982). Copper Iontophoresis in male contraception. *Andrologia*, **14**, 481
8. Settlage, D. S. F., March, C. M., Tredway, D. R., Umezaki, C. U. and Mishell, D. R., Jr. (1975). Effect of intrauterine device upon sperm transport in human female genital tract. *Gynecol. Invest.*, **6**, 2
9. Aref, I., Kandil, O., Tagi, A. El. and Morad, M. R. (1983). Effects of non-medicated and copper IUDs on sperm migration. *Contracept. Deliv. Syst.*, **4**, 203
10. Koch, U. J. (1980). Sperm migration in the human female genital tract with and without intrauterine devices. *Acta Europaea Fertilitatis*, **11**, 733
11. Smart, Y. C., Fraser, I. S., Clancy, R. L., Roberts, T. K. and Cripps, A. W. (1982). Early pregnancy factor as a monitor for fertilization in women wearing intrauterine devices. *Fertil. Steril.*, **37**, 201
12. Blandau, R. J. (1977). Comparative morphology and physiology of the cervix in several different animals and their relationship to sperm transport. In *The uterine cervix in reproduction*. Insler, V. and Bettendorf, G., eds. pp. 36–43. (Stuttgart: Georg Thieme Publishers)

25
Early chorionic activity in IUD bearing women. Preliminary report

L. VIDELA-RIVERO, S. BORTOLUSSI, J. J. ETCHEPAREBORDA
AND E. KESSERÜ

INTRODUCTION

The mechanism of the contraceptive action of intrauterine devices (IUDs) is not only incompletely understood at the present time, but is also rather controversial, in spite of the large amount of work done in this particular[1]. One possible mechanism could be an anti-implantatory effect of the fertilized egg. This has not yet been fully demonstrated[2], nevertheless it is being considered at the most likely, at least for the inert models. On the other hand, for the specific case of copper-bearing IUDs, there is mounting evidence[3,4] that the deleterious effect of copper ions on sperm vitality and migration may play an important role.

In this preliminary report the existence of early signs of implantation were investigated in the presence of inert as well as copper containing IUDs.

SUBJECTS

Forty-five women of child bearing age, with demonstrated fertility within the last 2 years, and showing biphasic menstrual cycles were studied. The women were divided into two groups, according to the type of IUD they had been fitted with: (a) inert IUD (Lippes Loop C) n = 27, and (b) copper IUD (Nova T) n = 18.

METHOD

The methodology followed in each cycle has been summarized in Figure 1.

Serial colpocytology and cervical mucus assessment were carried out to ascertain the ovulatory phase of the cycle. At a day closest to ovulation, a

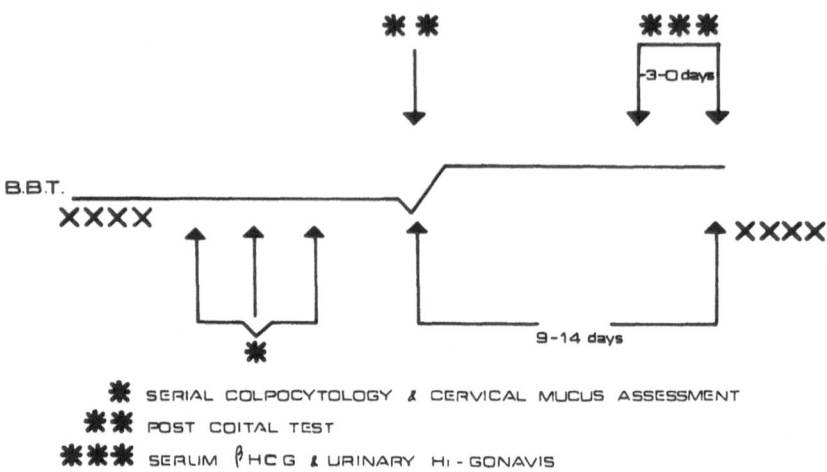

Figure 1 Methods. B.B.T.: Basal body temperature; × × × × : Days of menstruation; *: Serial colpocytology cervical and mucus assessment; **: Post-coital test; ***: Serum β-hCG and urinary Hi–Gonavis

post-coital test was done. Cycles which did not prove to be ovulatory or where the post-coital test did not show optimal values have been excluded from the study. In the remaining cycles, meeting all the requirements, the existence of early implantation signs were searched for 9–14 days after ovulation; i.e. 3–0 days before the next menses. The parameters measured were simultaneous serum β-hCG as well as urinary hCG determinations.

Serum β-hCG was measured by RIA, and urinary hCG by the early Hi––Gonavis method. The following indicative values for an early chorionic activity were considered: β-hCG fraction $\geqslant 10\,mUI/ml$ serum[5]; and urinary hCG $\geqslant 40\,IU/l$[6].

RESULTS

In the inert IUD group, in 4 out of 27 cases indicative values for early chorionic activity were detected. This is in contrast with the values shown by the copper IUD group in which there were no cases with those indicative values. Summarizing, premenstrual chorionic activity showed an incidence of 15% in the inert IUD group and 0% in the copper IUD group.

DISCUSSION

There is no doubt that the so-called 'early chorionic activity signs' has not yet been elucidated in terms of the actual existence of the implantation of a fertilized egg. On the other hand the low number of subjects in this preliminary report cannot be considered as conclusive, however, it seems that a difference between the inert and the copper-containing IUDs does exist, with a total absence of chorionic activity in the latter. This finding would be consistent with the anti-implantatory mechanism postulated for inert IUDs, and also with the sperm inhibiting mechanism suggested for the copper IUDs.

As the next step towards resolving this question, we have started to apply the same methodology to a third group of women who do not use any contraceptive method and who display apparently normal cycles but which do not result in actual pregnancy.

References

1. Tatum, H. J. (1977). Clinical aspect of intrauterine contraception. *Fertil. Steril.*, **28**, 3
2. Sagiroglu, N. and Sagiroglu, E. (1970). Biologic mode of actions of the lippes loop in intrauterine contraception. *Am. J. Obstet. Gynecol.*, **106**, 506
3. Kesserü, E. (1975). Influence of hormonal and intrauterine contraceptives on human sperm. In Hafez, E. S. E. and Thibault, C. G. (eds.) *The Biology of Spermatozoa.* pp. 239–49. (Basel: S. Karger)
4. Holland, M. K. and White, I. G. (1982). Heavy metals and human spermatozoa; II. The effect of seminal plasma on the toxicity of copper metal for spermatozoa. *Int. J. Fertil.*, **27**, 95
5. Lenton, E. A., Neal, L. M. and Sulaiman, R. (1982). Plasma concentrations of human chorionic gonadotropin from the time of implantation until the second week of pregnancy. *Fertil. Steril.*, **37**, 773
6. Tojo, N., Kanazawa, S., Maruo, T., Sanjo, K. and Sakagmi, A. (1973). Stimulation of low level hCG in urine by Hi–Gonavis. *Clin. Endocrinol. (Jpn)*, **21**, 1179

26
Cytological findings in women with different methods of fertility regulation including spermatozoal recovery rates

U. J. KOCH

An examination of the influence of the methods of contraception and menstrual hygiene on the cytological Pap. smears gave the following results. 1943 women were investigated, and data from the cytological results were documented by the 'Munich Scheme' according Soost and Baur (1980)[1], evaluated in two age-groups (21–35 and 36–50 years) and according to the manner of menstrual hygiene (tampons or pads). The majority of younger women used tampons. This group of women showed the largest proportion of Pap. smear group I. In the group of elder women the proportions of the Pap. smear groups were less favourable. The distribution shows that the results of Pap. smear group III (dubious) were three-fold higher. The results of Pap. smear group II (atypical, unsuspicious) were also increased in the group using tampons. The pad-users demonstrated the least favourable distribution in the cytological Pap. smear group statistical analysis. In all contraception groups the tampon-users of the younger women had the largest proportion of inconspicuous cytological results (Pap. smear group I). The proportion of Pap. smear group I of the users of the IUD ML Cu 250 amounted to 89.5%. This distribution was the most favourable of the whole study.

Only the younger users of pads in combination with spermicides and barrier methods showed an exception in the most unfavourable Pap. smear group distribution. The group of elder women showed comparable results.

In all groups the so-called pure Döderlein bacilli flora was seen only in every fourth woman. The majority of the investigated women presented a so-called bacterial mixed-flora, in 15% of these women *Candida albicans* and/or *Trichomonas vaginalis* were observed. The proportion of *Haemophilus (gardnerella) vaginalis* in the group with the bacterial mixed-flora amounted to 25%. Only for simplification, the group with Döderlein bacilli was contrasted to the combined bacterial mixed-flora group. In the younger contraception-group using spermicidal agents and barrier methods, the users of pads with the Pap. smear group I had the largest proportion of pure Döderlein bacilli flora (27.9%). The proportion of pure Döderlein bacilli flora was reduced in the group of women using oral contraceptives and of Pap. smear group I. As was expected, in the Pap. smear group II an almost total substitution of the pure Döderlein bacilli flora by the mixed bacterial flora took place; the proportion of vaginal leukocytosis was increased in Pap. smear group II; only in the Pap. smear group I, the younger women using oral contraceptives and tampons was an increased proportion of vaginal leukocytosis seen (54.4%). The women using the ML Cu 250 and the women with spermicides and barrier methods did not differ in vaginal or cervical leukocytosis. In the age-group of the older women a similar status was seen; in the group of the women with the IUD and Pap. smear group I the proportion of pure Döderlein bacilli flora was reduced, and the proportion with vaginal leukocytosis was increased in comparison to the younger women. The proportion of cervical leukocytosis seen amounted to only half that of vaginal leukocytosis. It could be established that in IUD bearing women there are no specific cytological changes, and that in these women the use of tampons could be recommended without hesitation.

The investigation of the influence of coital frequency in women using different methods of contraception on the cytological results led to the following findings: the mean monthly coital frequency was in both age-groups of IUD-bearing women the highest. In the group of younger women with the ML Cu 250 *in situ* it amounted to 11.3 and in the elder women to 8.6. The corresponding results in women using oral contraceptives were 8.5 and 5.5, and in women using spermicides and barrier methods 7.9 and 5.9. Although in IUD-bearing women no increase of cyto-pathological results could be observed, and although these women showed the highest monthly coital frequency, it could be established, that under these conditions an influence on the cervical cytology is not existent. These calculated data do not allow the conclusion to be drawn that the contraceptive method influences sexual activity, or that women with different degrees of sexual activity prefer particular methods of contraception; these factors are now being investigated.

The influence of the different methods of contraception on sperm migration in comparison to women with the desire for pregnancy was proved (Table 1). It was seen that in the case of a normal female genital tract and a fertile partner, around the day of ovulation, the cervical post-coital test according to Sims and Hühner[2] was positive in 70% of cases. In sterility work-ups, it was seen that

Table 1 Cervical postcoital test according to Sims and Hühner[2] (S.H.–T.) and peritoneal sperm migration test (P.S.M.–T.) according to Koch, Hammerstein and Zielske[3] in women without and with different methods of fertility regulation (n : 497)

	Cervical postcoital test (S.H.–T.) % positive results	Peritoneal sperm migration test (P.S.M.–T) % positive results
Women without contraception (with desire for pregnancy, normal female genital tract and fertile partner)	70	50
Women with contraception		
Rhythm method	20	not investigated
Coitus interruptus	16	not investigated
Barrier methods and spermicides	0	not investigated
Oral contraceptives		
sequential pills	36	(+)*
combination pills	3	0*
progestogen pills	(+)*	not investigated
Intrauterine devices		
inert IUDs	(+)*	(+)*
progesterone IUDs	(+)*	not investigated
copper IUDs (ML Cu 250)	21	0 (n : 50)

*Only a small number of investigated women

there is a direct correlation between spermatozoal recovery rates in the peritoneal fluid and the prognosis for later pregnancies. In normal functioning partners, after a single cohabitation around the day of ovulation, in 50% of the investigated women, spermatozoa could be detected in the peritoneal fluid after the first investigation. The highest pregnancy rates were seen where the cervical and peritoneal sperm migration tests were positive. In cases of negative cervical and peritoneal sperm migration tests and patent oviducts, pregnancies cannot be expected.

In women using the rhythm method, spermatozoa were found in 20% at the level of the uterine cervix around the day of ovulation. Also in women practising coitus interruptus, spermatozoa were recovered in 16%, but in women using the combination of barrier methods and spermicides in no case were spermatozoa detected in the preovulatory cervical mucus. These data are in agreement with the Pearl-indices for these contraceptive methods. In women using typical sequential oral contraceptives, sperm migration seems to be undisturbed in the first phase of treatment. However, in women using monophasic combination oral contraceptives, sperm migration was extremely inhibited, especially at the area of the uterine cervix due to the modified mucus by progestogens. In no case could spermatozoa be found in the peritoneal fluid of these women. In women bearing inert IUDs (Lippes Loop) sperm migration can normally be observed in the whole female genital tract. In contrast to inert-IUD users, an inhibition of sperm migration could be demonstrated in women bearing copper IUDs, especially the ML Cu 250, by cervical *in vivo* and *in vitro* sperm migration tests.

In 50 women, the peritoneal sperm migration test (PSM-Test[3]) was performed, when the IUD ML Cu 250 was in place. Although in these women the cervical post-coital tests[2] around the day of ovulation were positive, no spermatozoa could be detected in the peritoneal fluid (Figure 1). Elimination of spermatozoa takes place in the entire female genital tract by macrophages and the polymorphonuclear leukocytes[4,5].

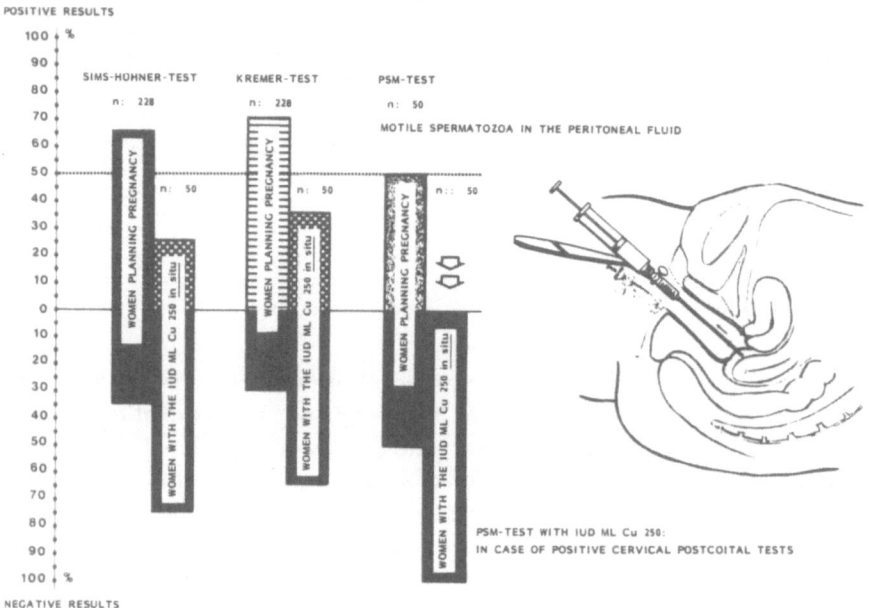

Figure 1 Post-coital test (according to Sims-Hühner[2a,b]), sperm migration test (according to Kremer[7]) and peritoneal sperm migration test (PSM-Test according to Koch, Hammerstein and Zielske[3]) without and with the copper bearing IUD ML Cu 250 *in situ*

A partial effect in the multifactorial mode of action of copper bearing IUDs seems to be the inhibition of transtubal sperm migration, which is a parameter of fertility. The endometrial foreign body reaction, caused by the copper IUD inhibits or blocks transtubal sperm migration, due to an increased phagocytosis of spermatozoa by the increase in leukocytes[6]. The influences on the blastocyst are of minor importance in the mode of copper IUD-action, because according to our opinion, in cases of disturbed sperm migration, fertilization does not occur.

References

1. Soost, H. J. and Baur, S. (1980). *Gynaekologische Zytodiagnostik*. (Stuttgart-New York: Thieme)
2a. Sims, J. M. (1866). Clinical notes on uterine surgery. (New York: W. Wood)
2b. Hühner, M. (1913). Sterility in the male and female and its treatment. (New York: Rebman Co.)
3. Koch, U. J., Zielske, F. and Hammerstein, J. (1974). Nachweis der Spermatozoenaszension im weilblichen Genitaltrakt als Routineuntersuchng in der Sterilitätsdiagnostik. *Arch. Gynäk.*, **219**, 610
4. Koch, U. J. and Vogel, M. (1981). Leukocytes and their influence on sperm migration in the human female genital tract including the peritoneal cavity. *Proceedings of the III World Congress on Human Reproduction*. p. 501. (Amsterdam: Excerpta Medica)
5. Koch, U. J. (1980). Sperm migration in the human female genital tract with and without intrauterine devices. *Acta Eur. Fertil.*, **11**, 733
6. Sagiroglu, N. and Sagiroglu, E. (1970). The cytology of intrauterine contraceptive devices. *Acta Cytol.*, (Baltimore), **14**, 58
7. Kremer, J. (1965). A simple sperm penetration test. *Int. J. Fertil.*, **10**, 209

27
A bacteriological study of the endometrial cavity, after up to seven years use of butterfly IUD

H. G. MASSOURAS, E. KOUMENDAKOU, Z. DELATOLA
AND V. FRYGANA

INTRODUCTION

The 'normal flora' may be described as a varied group of organisms that colonize a given area in a host without causing disease. Döderlein in 1892 first described the microbial flora of the female genital tract.

Many authors have found the following organisms, but in different percentages, in the genital tract (vagina and cervix) of healthy adult women[1,2]:

(1) Lactobacilli (also reported as Döderlein's Bacilli) in more than 70%,
(2) *Staphylococcus epidermitis* and diphtheroids, 30–60%,
(3) α-haemolytic streptococci, 16–53%,
(4) β-haemolytic streptococci, 1.6–27%,
(5) Non-haemolytic streptococci, 4.3–33%,
(6) Group D streptococci, 9.6–41.4%, and
(7) *Escherichia coli*, 3.3–28%.

The non-pregnant uterine cavity is nearly always considered to be sterile[3], although there is some controversy[4]. For many centuries Arab camel owners have used foreign bodies (e.g. round stones) as an IUD for contraception. It was about 1878 that intrauterine devices or stem pessaries were first used for contraception in humans, and Dickinson in 1916 predicted that a simple intrauterine pessary would become a standard method of conception control. Since then many authors (Grafenberg 1928, Ota 1934) have described results of IUD contraception, but the serious side effects (including deaths) put the IUD out of use. In 1959 there appeared reports (Ishihama and Oppenheimer) on IUD contraception as a result of better hygienic conditions, the new shape and material of IUDs and use of antibiotics.

Since 1969 we have used the Massouras' Duck's Foot-IUD (MDF-IUD) and the Butterfly-IUD (Reweco Ltd, Athens, Greece) (Figures 1 and 2). We have had

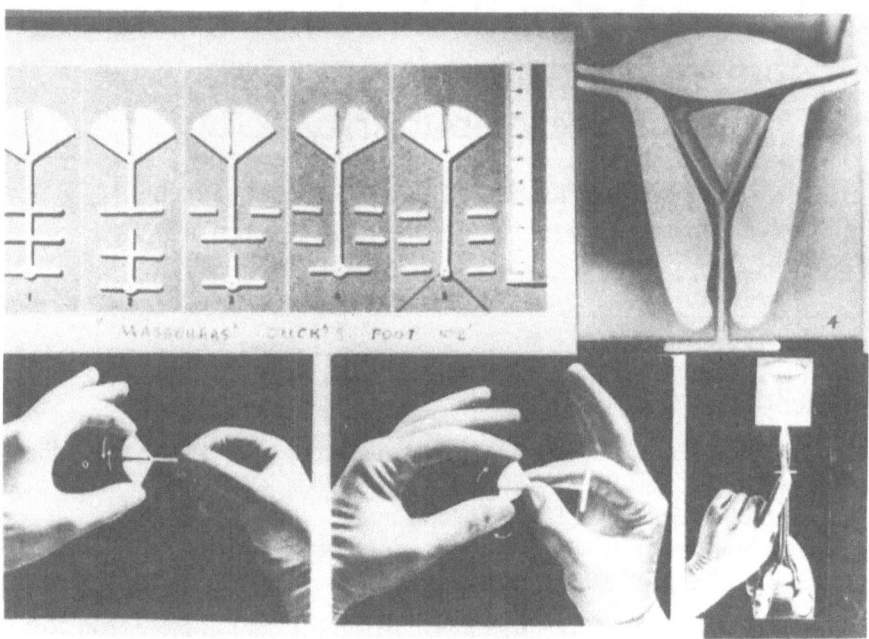

Figure 1 Massouras' Duck's Foot IUD – structure and method of insertion

very good results with these when correctly placed in uterine cavity because of the shape and material (inert polyethylene with barium sulphate for detection)[5, 6]. They consist of two triangular very fine wings, that completely cover the whole uterine cavity without any possibility of perforation, pregnancy or expulsion. Due to the special shape, the inert material and the very fine thickness of the wings of the IUD, which fill the normal uterine cavity without any pressure on the anterior and posterior surface of the uterus or the endometrium[7] we have noticed no significant difference in endometrial dating, and no cases of squamous metaplasia or endometritis have been seen.

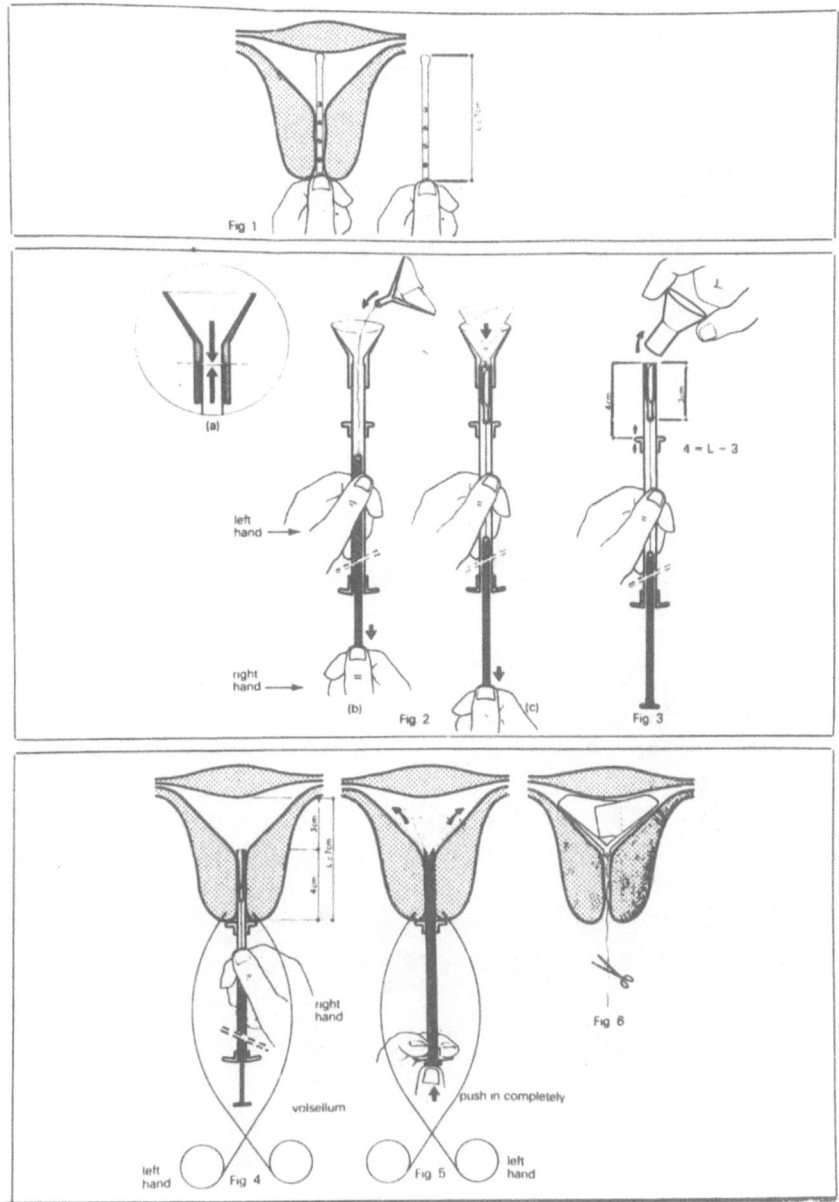

Figure 2 Butterfly IUD – method of insertion

MATERIAL AND METHODS

Cultures (aerobic, anaerobic and for mycoplasmas) were obtained from 50 women with a MDF-IUD (22 women) or a Butterfly-IUD (28 women) fitted for 1 month to 7 years without any untoward symptoms. The cultures were taken:

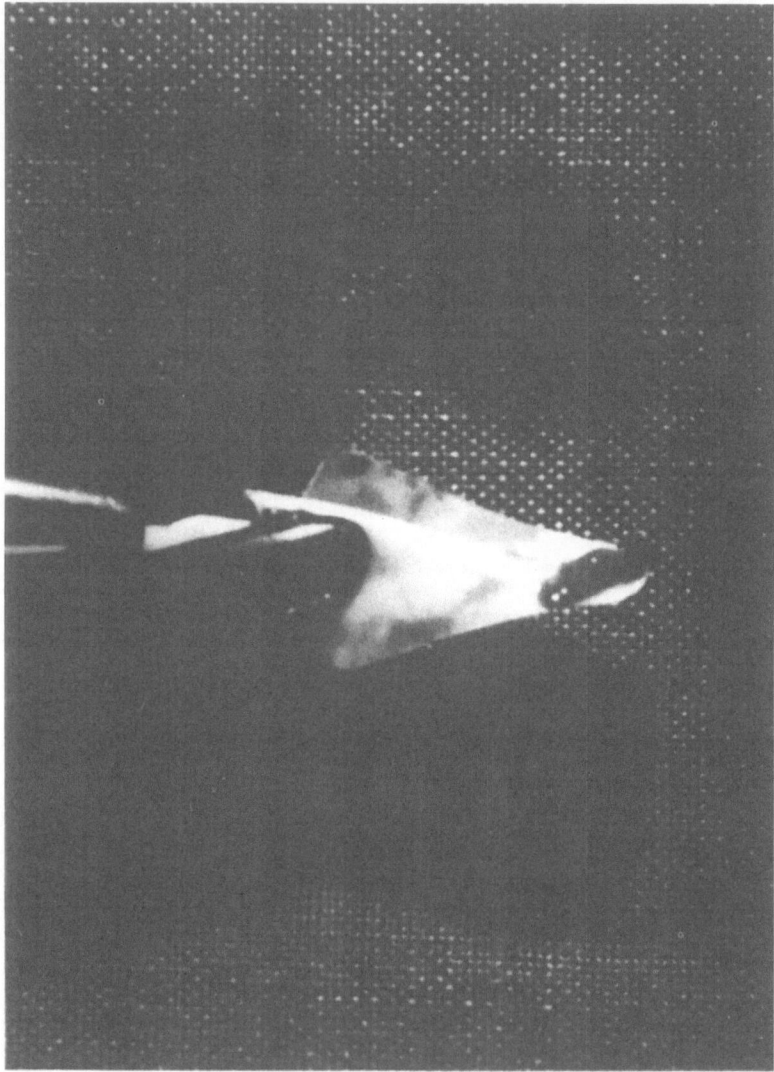

Figure 3 Butterfly IUD at the time of extraction. Notice that the two wings are rolled together keeping the internal surface of both wings (containing material from the endometrium) protected from contamination, as it is extracted through the endocervix

(1)   From the upper vagina through a special speculum,
(2)   From the endocervix after cleansing the exocervix with sterile gauze, and
(3)   From the internal surface between the two wings of the IUD (representing the endometrium), Figures 3 and 4.

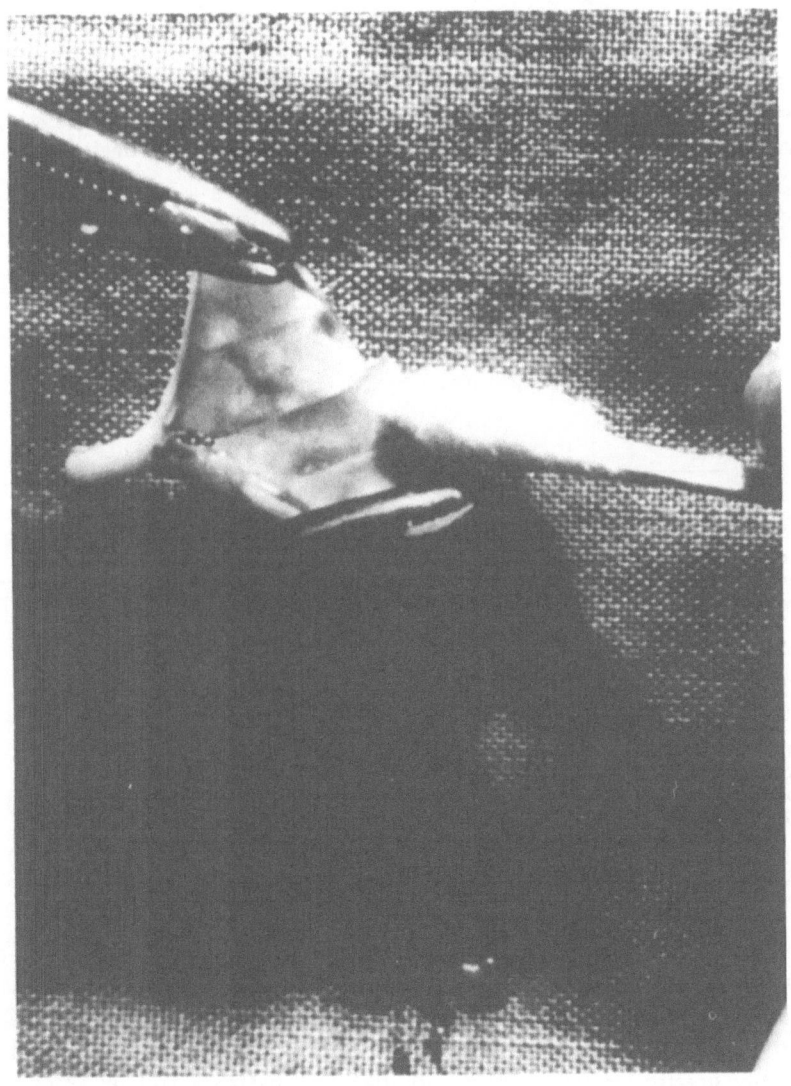

Figure 4   Method of taking a specimen for culture

157

The age of these women ranged from 22 to 42 years old, 80% were married, 12% single and 8% divorced. All of them had at least one D and C (after the last one the IUD was inserted), 85% of them had one child by caesarean section or natural childbirth. The frequency of coitus per week ranged from one up to six or unknown (the latter mostly among the single or divorced women).

RESULTS

In Table 1, we can see that in 31 out of 50 women (62%), the culture was positive, (a) vaginal culture, 16 cases (32%), (b) vaginal and endocervix, 12 (24%), and (c) vaginal and endocervix and IUD, 3 (6%). Table 2 shows the bacterial species

Table 1   Positive or negative cultures from vagina, endocervix and IUD

Women with IUD	Numbers	%
Positive	31	62
Vagina	16	32
Vagina and endocervix	12	24
Vagina + endocervix + IUD	3	6
Negative	19	38
Total	50	100

Table 2   Microbes isolated in positive cultures from vagina, endocervix and IUD, in 31 women with IUD *in situ*

Microbes	Vagina	Endocervix	IUD	Total
Candida sp.	5	5	2	12
Trichomonas	4	—	—	4
Ureaplasma urealyticum	21	2	—	23
Mycoplasma hominis	7	2	—	9
Streptococcus sp.	2	3	—	5
Peptostreptococcus	4	2	—	6
E. coli	4	2	—	6
Klebsiella aerogenes	1	2	1	4
Total	48	18	3	69

and their incidence isolated from the different areas, i.e. vagina, endocervix and IUD. Table 3 shows the parity of the women with the IUD *in situ* in relationship to the bacteriological findings. It is noteworthy that the greatest number of positive cultures was among the single or divorced women with no children, probably greater sexual activity with different partners and/or among the married women without children (where an hormonal imbalance probably existed) rather than among the married women with children. It appears that

Table 3 Relationship between the number of previous pregnancies and presence of microbes in IUD wearers

Number of natural childbirths, caesarean sections, D and C	Positive	Negative
0	14	5
1	5	—
2	2	3
3	2	3
4	3	5
5	3	—
6	2	—
7	—	—
8	—	3
Total	31	19

$p > 0.1$

as parity increases, so the number of positive cultures decreases possibly as the woman ages and after a number of pregnancies her libido diminishes. Although the above suggestion looks reasonable, it does not completely agree with Table 4.

Table 4 Relationship between frequency of coitus per week and presence of pathogenic microbes in IUD wearers

Coitus per week	Positive	Negative
1	3	—
2	3	2
3	10	5
4	5	2
5	—	3
6	—	3
>6	2	—
unknown	8	4
Total	31	19

$p > 0.1$

We can see from Scheme 1 that the positive cultures have an inverse relationship to the duration of insertion of the IUD i.e. when the number of positive cultures is high the time is short and when the positive cultures are low the time is long (as many other authors have noticed).

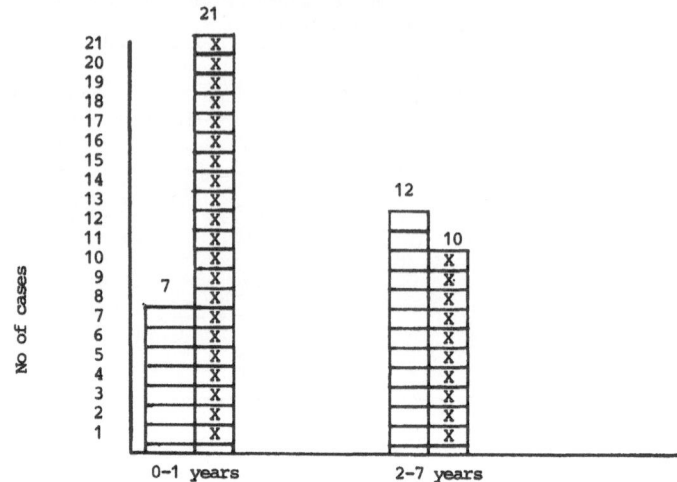

Scheme 1 Relationship between length of time of IUD *in situ* and presence of pathogens (X = positive for pathogens) (*p* < 0.1)

Table 5 Patient data and pathogens isolated from three IUD users

Patient	Age and marital status	Pregnancies and D and C	Frequency of coitus/week	Duration of IUD use	Cultures
S.V.	31 married	3 preg 1 D and C	3–5	10 months	IUD *Candida* sp. Endocervix *Candida* sp. Vagina *Candida* sp. *U. urealyticum*
K.E.	35 married	primary infertility	1–3	6 weeks	IUD *Kl. aerogenes* Endocervix *Kl. aèrogenes* Vagina *Kl. aerogenes*
P.A.	32 married	primary infertility	1–3	2 weeks	IUD *Candida* sp. Endocervix *Candida* sp. Vagina *Candida* sp. *U. urealyticum*

CONCLUSIONS

Table 5 shows data from three patients having positive IUD cultures. As can be seen the *in situ* time was too short in all cases.

Secondly, as we know *Candida albicans* and *Klebsiella aerogenes* are both micro-organisms of low virulence, needing a defective local or general resistance to produce infection. Therefore, we should look for these factors as a cause of these infections rather than to blame the IUD itself.

And indeed in these three women we did find a lowering of the general and local resistance. Only the first woman (s.v.) was healthy and had children. The other two had an hormonal imbalance and came to us for treatment of primary infertility. One of these patients had been operated on twice for cystic ovaries and she only had one third of a single ovary remaining at that time; the other, had an hypoplastic uterus with hormonal imbalance.

Finally, we could say that the IUD culture in a healthy normal uterus should be considered as negative.

ACKNOWLEDGEMENT

I would like to thank the staff of the microbiological laboratory at Aretaion hospital, particularly Dr E. Filippopoulou who was responsible for the anaerobic cultures and Dr L. Kouskouni who was responsible for the myco-plasma cultures, for their help and co-operation in this study.

References

1. Galask, R. P., Larsen, B. and Ohm, M. J. (1976). Vaginal flora and its role in disease entities. *Clin. Obstet. Gynecol.*, **19**, 61
2. Koumendakou, E., Filippopoulou, E., Kourkouli E., Kouskouni, E. and Sykiotis, C. (1982). Genital Mycoplasmas in Vaginitis. *Acta Microbiol. Hellen.*, **27**, 178–87
3. Mishell, D. R., Bell, J. H., Good, R. G. and Moyer, D. L. (1966). The intrauterine device: A bacteriologic study of the endometrial cavity. *Am. J. Obstet. Gynecol.*, **96**, 119
4. Willson, J. R., Bollinger, Ch. C. and Leder, W. J. (1964). The effect of an intrauterine contra-ceptive device on the bacterial flora of the endometrial cavity. *Am. J. Obstet. Gynecol.*, **20**, 726
5. Massouras, H. G. (1973). Intra-uterine adhesions: A syndrome of the past with the use of the "Massouras Duck's Foot No. 2, Intra Uterine Contraceptive Device". *Am. J. Obstet. Gynecol.*, **4**, 576–8
6. Massouras, H. G., Coutifaris, B. and Kalogirou, D. (2nd University Clinic of Athens) (1982). Management of uterine adhesions with "Massouras' Duck's Foot" and "Butterfly" IUDs. In *Contracept. Deliv. Syst.*, **3**, 25–38.
7. Massouras, H. G., Papaharalambous, N., Kyroudi, A. and Voulgaris, Z. (1979). Histological findings of Endometrium in women with Massouras' Duck's Foot IUD *in situ*. *Proceedings of the 1st International Symposium of Medicated IUD and Polymeric Delivery Systems*, June 28–30, Amsterdam

28
The IUD: a decade review

R. SNOWDEN

The UK IUD Research Network which holds the greatest amount of IUD data in the United Kingdom was officially set up in 1971, and since that time the experiences of tens of thousands of women have been carefully monitored. During the last decade intrauterine devices have come and gone, some have disappeared with hardly a trace, whilst the going of others has been heralded by legal infighting involving untold millions of dollars. What happened to the Latex Leaf, the Birnberg Bow, the LEM, Ahmed's Device (or the Hong Kong Triangle) and the stainless steel M Device (the M211 and M213) with and without a Teflon coating? These and others are either no longer with us or are fitted in such few numbers that they are no longer of international relevance. The most well publicised device that met its end during the last decade was the Dalkon Shield, perhaps more sinned against than sinning.

In their place has come the Gravigard or Cu 7, the Gyne T (Cu T), the Progestasert, the Multiload ML Cu 250 and the Novagard. Our old friend from the 1960s – the Lippes Loop – is still with us, but its smaller sizes are seldom fitted and sales of its major competitor in Europe, the Saf-T-Coil has just recently been discontinued in the United Kingdom. Nostalgia to an enthusiast provides a gentle sense of satisfaction, but times change and the new must replace the old. But why? The obvious answer is that with progress comes greater efficiency and effectiveness, but sometimes this is hard to discern when examining the development of IUDs. In the 1930s Grafenberg, that great IUD pioneer, was demonstrating a pregnancy rate with his device of between one and two women in every hundred during each year of use. With more sophisticated IUDs and whole departments of statisticians providing statistical tables that keep computers busy for hours, the pregnancy rate for most IUDs in the 1980s remains almost identical to that presented by Grafenberg just 50 years

163

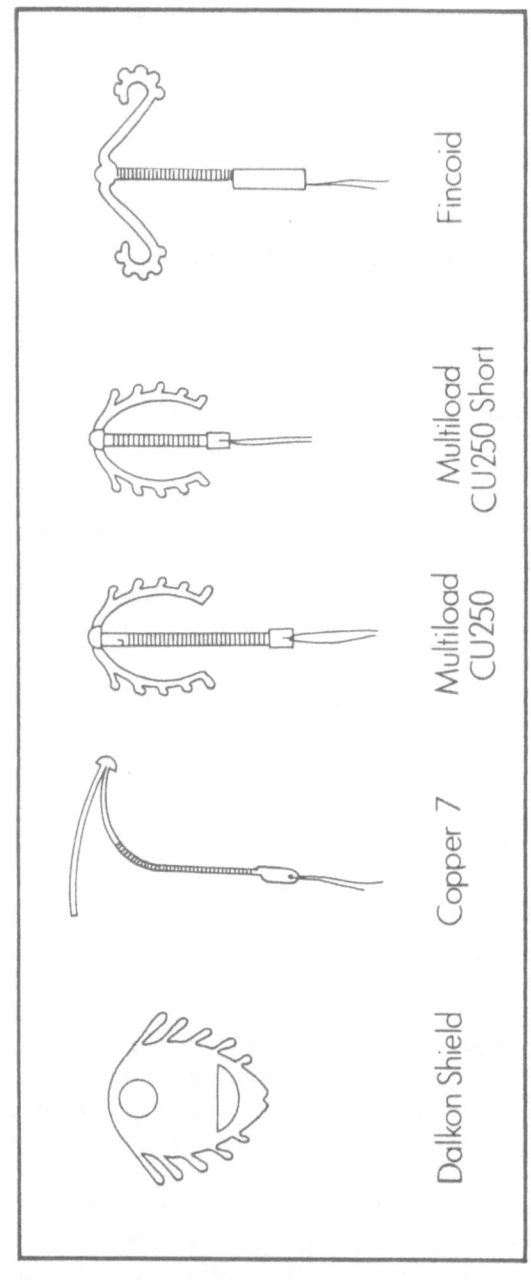

Figure 1

ago. Fads and fashions in IUD design, like the IUDs themselves, come and go, sometimes with little evidence of the new being an advance over the old.

For the purposes of this brief idiosyncratic review, one relatively new device, the Multiload Cu 250 being of recent European origin, is taken as an example of IUD development to demonstrate changes in IUD design and use during the last 10 years. Like most modern IUDs, this device did not arrive spontaneously, its size, shape and composition owe much to the IUDs that preceded it. The influence of the Dalkon Shield with its five lateral fins and also of the Cu 7 are obvious. It is also of interest to note how the ML 250 has itself led to further refinements both within the model itself and for other models developed by other, presumably competing, manufacturers (Figure 1).

IUD FITTING

To be of use, an IUD must be fitted into the right place with a minimum of discomfort to the IUD wearer; it should prevent pregnancy, resist expulsion and avoid the creation of unwanted side effects necessitating its removal, and it should be capable of removal when this is desired, again without undue discomfort or inconvenience to the IUD user. Unfortunately, these ideal conditions often conflict. A device that is easy to fit tends to expel more easily, and a higher rate of expulsion is linked to a higher rate of pregnancy. Similarly, a device that is easy to remove is also more likely to be expelled during use.

At a more personal level for the IUD fitting doctor, ease of IUD fitting may even be counter-productive. The paradoxical situation whereby ease of fitting is related to incorrect placing of the device leading to early expulsion and possible pregnancy is not unknown. The experience of the teams in the UK IUD Research Network suggest that there is less variability *between doctors* when more care has to be taken in fitting the IUD when compared to devices that are fitted without the need for such care. An IUD, it seems, not only has to cope with possible experiences relating to the IUD user; apart from being 'patient proof' the device and its fitting must also be 'doctor proof'. If an IUD can be incorrectly fitted it *will* be so fitted. What is needed then is not a device that merely provides a low pregnancy rate, but one that minimizes the probability of difficulty across a range of possible events associated with the IUD user and the person responsible for IUD fitting. One aspect of IUD fitting that has been debated in recent years is the use of a tenaculum to pull the uterus into line with the cervical canal. With IUD inserters consisting of an outer sleeve and an internal plunger (all of the devices utilizing a small bore inserter), two hands are required; one to hold the outer sleeve of the inserter and the other to operate the internal plunger which either pushes the device into the uterus or leaves it there by retracting the outer sleeve over the plunger. A third hand is then required to manipulate the tenaculum. A device which is fitted by using a hollow tube without an internal plunger, may be more bulky to pass through the cervical canal but correct alignment of the cervical canal and uterus is easier to maintain.

IUD EXPULSION

Once in the uterus, the IUD is expected to stay there. Some devices have been specifically designed to make expulsion difficult. The stainless steel 'M' devices were just such devices, and the Dalkon Shield with its fundal seeking characteristics was another. The similarity in the shape of the Multiload IUD to the Dalkon Shield indicates that a low expulsion rate would be expected with the new device, and this has been borne out in a number of studies. For general programme reasons it may be more efficient to use a device which, although inconvenient to fit, also has a low rate of expulsion. This is especially relevant among a population that is reluctant or unable to return to the medical facility for regular follow-up visits.

IUD PREGNANCY

Pregnancy rates are linked to the rate of expulsion, and both of these are associated with the age and parity of the IUD wearer. Having said this, the differences between devices remains small, though this can be of little support to the IUD user who becomes pregnant. Most devices in general use give an annual pregnancy rate of less that 2 per 100 women per year.

IUD REMOVAL

The single most common reason for known IUD discontinuation is that associated with removal of the device resulting from complaints of excess bleeding and/or abdominal pain. It is also known that the interpretation and treatment of these side effects depend as much upon personal and social factors affecting both the IUD user and the person to whom she may complain. Of all the side effects of IUD use, these are the ones which vary most according to non-medically defined factors. Attempts are being made to develop IUDs which release hormones directly into the uterus with the aim of reducing the amount and duration of bleeding, but these belong to the next decade review. It seems that a device which reduces the likelihood of displacement or expulsion, but is also flexible enough to avoid unacceptable levels of bleeding, has been a useful development in the decade just completed.

THE IUD AND INFECTION

During the 1970s, the incidence of infection among IUD users has become a matter of major concern. Whilst not experiencing the same rate of infection for some devices as reported in the USA, a detailed analysis of the UK data indicates that a small risk (about 1 woman in every 100 each year) does exist, no IUD consistently demonstrates that it is worse or better than other IUDs in relation to reported infection. Reports of actinomycoses-like organisms found among IUD users have been made, but these findings have not been of such magnitude to warrant IUD removal on a routine basis. Septic spontaneous abortion among pregnant IUD users has not been a feature of the UK IUD experience, although some cases are believed to have occurred.

IUD AND THE THE USE OF COPPER

One significant step during the last decade has been in the inclusion of copper as an anti-fertility agent, either in the form of fine wire or solid sleeves which is attached to the body of the IUD. Like other fashions in IUD design there are the supporters and occasional detractors of this development. Whilst some evidence points to a reduction in the pregnancy rate when copper is added to the IUD body, other evidence indicates that no such avoidance of pregnancies actually takes place. One interesting finding has been that copper IUDs worn for lengthy periods of time do not appear to be associated with an increase in the pregnancy rate. The assumption that pregnancy rates will rise as the release of copper ions diminishes, owing to the copper being expended, has not been borne out by clinical experience. The debate surrounding the usefulness of copper will, no doubt, continue.

CONCLUSIONS

The last ten years experience in the UK IUD Research Network indicates:

(1) Pregnancy rates have not significantly altered, despite changes in IUD design.
(2) Expulsion rates have fallen as new devices such as the Multiload have been introduced.
(3) Removal of IUDs following a complaint of bleeding and/or pain have tended to fall.
(4) There is a greater effect of age and parity than at first appreciated.
(5) There is often a greater variation between IUD fitting centres than between IUD models.
(6) Examination of the interaction of the events associated with pregnancy, expulsion and removal is a more realistic approach as compared to the assessment of the pregnancy rate alone.

(7) A flexible device resistant to expulsion will generally be more successful than other devices, despite some possible discomfort at fitting and removal.

(8) The inclusion of copper to the body of the IUD has not resulted in a reduction in the pregnancy rate when compared to the rates obtained using other devices that do not carry copper.

The Multiload IUD

The Multiload is an IUD that requires care in fitting, but is generally resistant to expulsion. This device has the lowest rate of expulsion for any device currently fitted in the UK IUD Research Network (Table 1). The Multiload has a moderate rate of removal following complaints of bleeding or pain and, in common with other IUDs, has a low pregnancy rate. As far as IUD programmes are concerned what is needed is a device which is difficult to expel, is flexible enough to reduce undue bleeding, can be fitted in parous women who may not return for regular follow-up visits, and is capable of reducing variance in expulsion rates between IUD-fitting doctors. In all these aspects of IUD use the Multiload demonstrates an advance in IUD design resulting in the arrival of a serious European competitor in a market dominated by American manufacturers.

Table 1 Selected gross cumulative rates for the Multiload (ML 250), Gravigard (Cu 7) and Lippes Loop C among parous women to 12 months of use per 100 users*

	ML 250	LL C	Cu 7
Pregnancy	1.7 (0.7–3.3)	1.1 (0.8–1.4)	2.0 (1.7–2.3)
Expulsion	4.9 (3.1–6.8)	6.4 (5.7–7.0)	9.7 (9.1–10.3)
Removal (bleeding/pain)	10.3 (7.7–13.0)	10.8 (9.9–11.8)	9.9 (9.3–10.6)
No. of women	656	5952	11 213
Months of observation	9491	51 155	95 588

Figures in brackets represent upper and lower limits at 95% confidence level computed using life table techniques
*These data were obtained from non-randomized field trials among a total of 17 821 women attending clinics in the UK IUD Research Network

Section 4

Abortion and Sterilization

29
Study on the effect of LH–RH analog in the termination of pregnancy

Y. YAOI, T. KUBOTA, H. OIYAMA, A. TEH, N. NISHI,
A. SUZUKI, M. SAITO, T. OHKURA, T. KUMASAKA
AND A. ARIMURA

While conducting studies on the induction of ovulation in anovulation, and the stimulation of luteal function in luteal insufficiency, with the hyperpotent analog of LH–RH, we found that the LH–RH analog was effective in inhibiting the gonadal functions. We therefore started studies on the possible use of the analog in the termination of early pregnancy and to investigate its mechanism of action. As a trial agent, we used [des-gly^{10}][pro^9-ethylamide]-LH–RH or D-leu^6-LH–RH-EA. Low levels of urinary hCG were measured by the Hi–Gonavis method.

In one case, the patient was 29 years old with secondary amenorrhoea, ovulation was induced by HMG and the luteal function was stimulated with hCG and superpotent analog [des-gly^{10}][pro^9-ethylamide]-LH–RH. But after the use of LH–RH analog, the serum progesterone levels gradually decreased, and several days later genital bleeding occurred. In another cycle, after ovulation by HMG, the luteal function was stimulated by hCG but urinary hCG levels did not increase, and it was suspected that implantation of the fertilized egg did not occur and late genital bleeding was seen. In the following year, i.e. January, 1970, pregnancy was diagnosed and by administration of the LH–RH analog, genital bleeding occurred. In another pregnancy in June, 1979, the analog was not used but hCG was given and the pregnancy progressed to term delivery. In this case, we recognized that the analog did not stimulate the luteal function, but it was luteolytic (Figure 1).

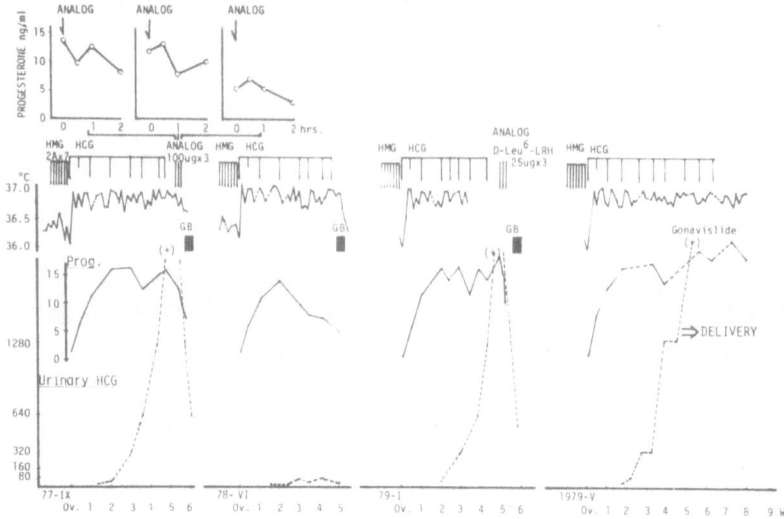

Figure 1 The changes of B.B.T. and serum hormonal levels after the administration of LH–RH analog, [des-gly^{10}][pro^9-ethylamide]-LH–RH, in early pregnancy following the induced ovulation

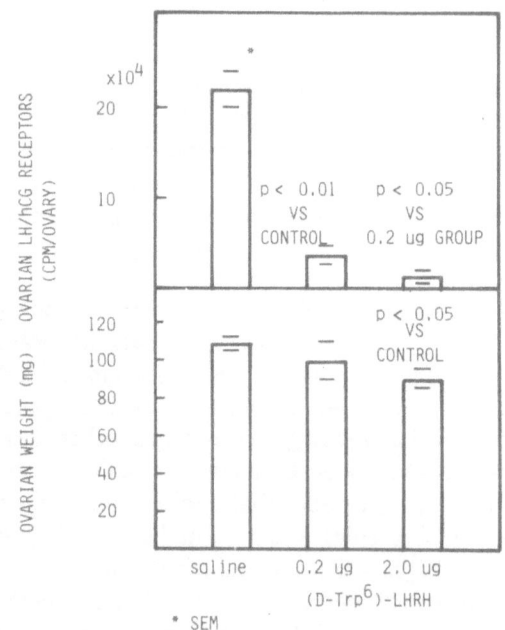

Figure 2 Effect of different doses of [D-Trp^6]-LH–RH on ovarian LH/hCG receptors of hypophysectomized immature rats pretreated with PMS (3 IU)

172

We called this characteristic of the LH–RH analog the 'paradoxical effect'. Then we studied the influence of the LH–RH analog on the gonadotropin receptors of the ovaries in rats. 0.2 μg and 2.0 μg of [D-trp⁶]-LH–RH signifi- cantly suppressed the ovarian LH/hCG receptors of hypophysectomized im- mature rats pretreated with PMS (Figure 2).

In 33 cases of women who were suspected of being pregnant and wanted termination of the pregnancy, the analog was given daily. In early stages of pregnancy (urinary hCG levels below 1000 IU/l), the administration of the analog disturbed the progress of the pregnancy and abortion took place in 11–13 cases within 7.2 days. However, if the analog was administered at later stages, the pregnancy could not be interrupted. When the treatment was started at the 6th week of gestation, 2–11 cases aborted within 7.5 days. At the 7th week, only 1–9 cases aborted within 10.0 days (Figure 3).

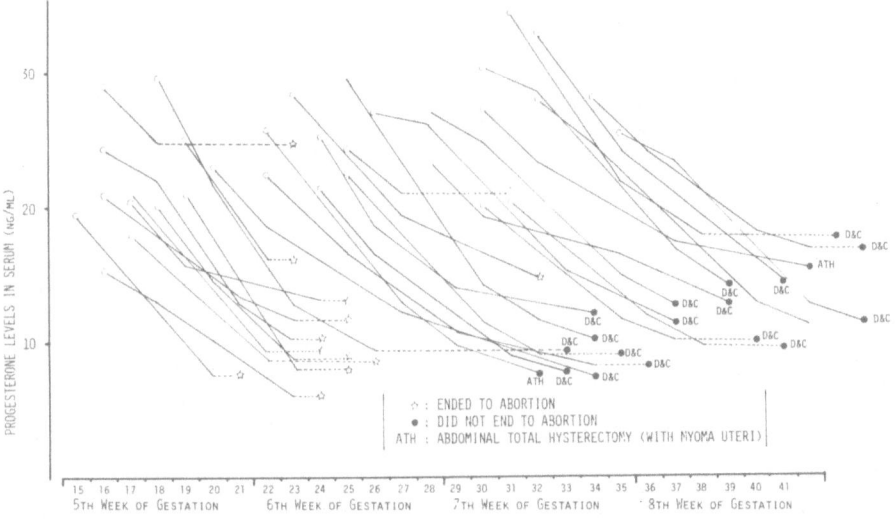

Figure 3 The influence of daily administration of agonistic analog of LH–RH on serum progesterone levels and on pregnancy

In the cases of myoma uteri combined with pregnancy, the analog was administered daily in the pre-operative period, and progesterone receptor levels in the removed uterine wall were measured. Progesterone receptors were signifi- cantly decreased by the daily administration of LH–RH analog (Figure 4).

The influence of the LH–RH analog and hCG on uterine weight was studied in rats. In the 15 day gestation group, after the injection of saline, uterine weights were 1.964 ± 0.409 g. And after the injection of LH–RH analog for the

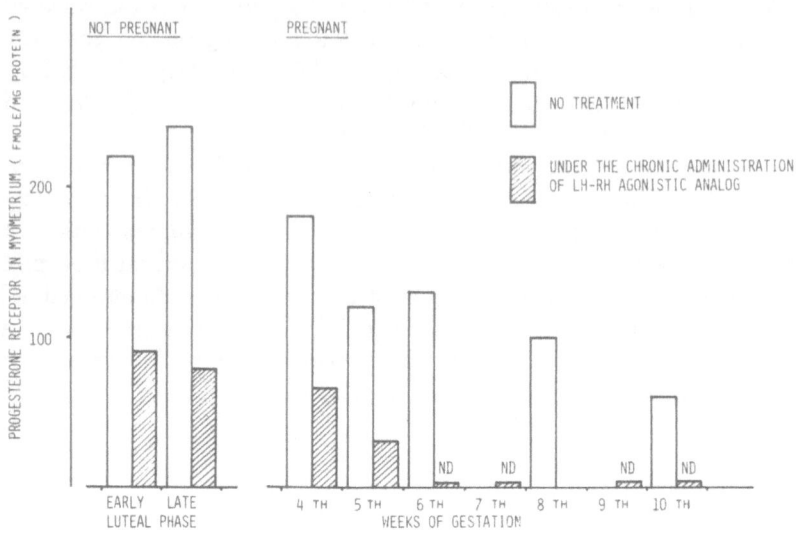

Figure 4 The influence of chronic administration of LH–RH agonistic analog on the progesterone receptor in myometrium in luteal phase and in early pregnancy

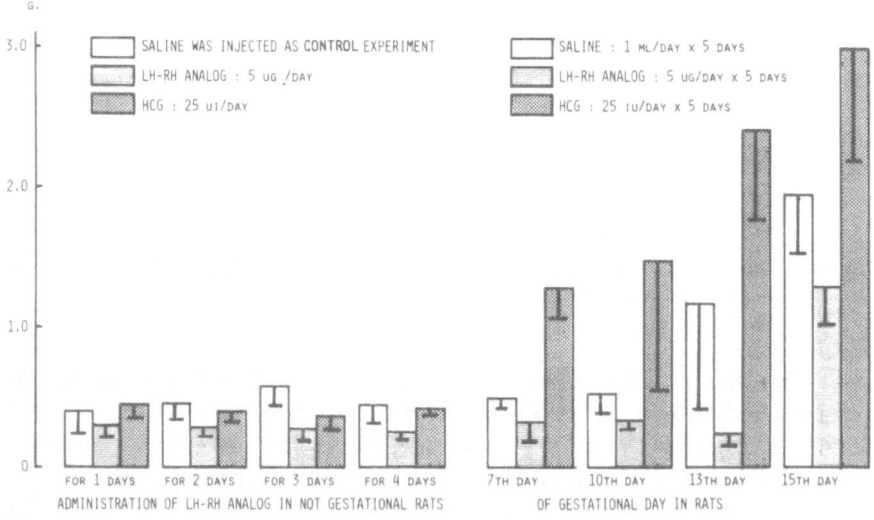

Figure 5 The influence of last 5 days administration LH–RH agonistic analog for uterine weight in early gestation in rats.

174

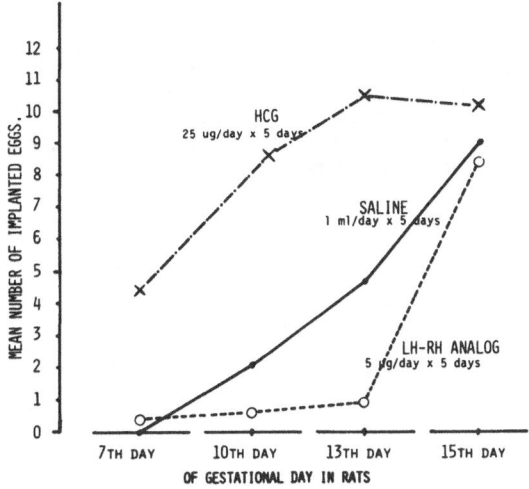

Figure 6 The influence of last 5 days administration of LH–RH agonistic analog and hCG for the implanted eggs in early gestation in rats

last 5 days 1.209 ± 0.246 g and after hCG 3.066 ± 0.799 g. In another group of 13 days gestation, uterine weights were 1.182 ± 0.987 g after saline, 0.268 ± 0.073 g after the LH–RH analog, and 2.422 ± 0.622 g after hCG. Daily administration for the last 5 days with the analog, suppressed the increase of uterine weight in gestational rats, especially in the early stages of gestation, but hCG, on the contrary, stimulated the development of uterine weights (Figure 5).

The numbers of implanted eggs were significantly changed, and the analog disturbed or dissolved the implanted eggs in the early stages of gestation, but it did not influence the progress of late stages of gestation. On the contrary, hCG stimulated the development of the implanted eggs (Figure 6).

These data suggested that the LH–RH analog inhibited not only the gonadotropin receptors of the ovary directly, but also disturbed the progesterone receptors in the uterine wall, thus interfering in the normal progress of early pregnancy and resulting in abortion. However, in the later stages of pregnancy, the effect of the analog was not strong enough to interfere with the pregnancy. We feel that the analog is an effective post coital contraceptive.

References

1. Saito, M., Kumasaka, T., Yaoi, Y., Nishi, N., Arimura, A., Coy, D. H. and Schally, A. V. (1977). Stimulation of LH and FSH secretion by (D-leu^6,des-gly^{10}-NH$_2$)-LH-RH-ethylamide after SC, Intravaginal and Intrarectal administration to women. *Fertil. Steril.*, **28**, 240–5
2. Yaoi, Y., Kumasaka, T., Nishi, N., Koyama, T., Ohkura, T., Saito, M., Arimura, A. and Scgally, S. V. (1976). Clinicial studies on Inducing Ovulation with [Des-Gly^{10}][Pro^9-ethylamide]-LH-RH, *5th International Congress of Endocrinology*, Hamburg

3. Yaoi, Y., Kubota, T., Imakita, T., Suzuki, A., Nishi, N., Teh, A., Ohkura, T., Koyama, T., Nishi, N., Saito, M., Kumasaka, T. and Arimura, A. (1980). Study on Induction of Ovulation by LH–RH Analog, *Xth International Congress of Fertility & Sterility*. Madrid
4. Bergquist, C., Nillius, S. J. and Wide, L. (1982). Long-term intranasal luteinizing hormone-releasing hormone agonist treatment for contraception in women. *Fertil. Steril.*, **38**, 190–3
5. Yen S. S. C. (1983). Clinical applications of gonadotropin-releasing hormone and gonadotropin-releasing hormone analogs. *Fertil. Steril.*, **39**, 257–66

30
Prophylactic metronidazole in first-trimester induced abortion. A clinical, controlled trial in high-risk women

L. HEISTERBERG AND K. PETERSEN

The most frequent complication following induced first-trimester abortion is pelvic infection. In a previous controlled, clinical trial testing the efficacy of prophylactic penicillin G and pivampicillin it was found that women with a history of pelvic inflammatory disease (PID) carried a significant risk (22%) of contracting a pelvic infection after abortion. The prophylactic treatment which significantly reduced this risk to 2% was administered for a total of 4 days. Additionally, women at gestational age 11–12 weeks were found to have an increased risk of post-abortal pelvic infection.

The purposes of the present study were: (1) to assess if short term prophylaxis with metronidazole alone would result in a clinical significant reduction of the post-abortal infection rate; (2) to confirm that women with previous PID were at risk; and (3) to demonstrate if other groups of women carried increased risks of postabortal infection.

Women referred to two gynaecological departments in Copenhagen for legal first-trimester abortions and who had a history of PID were asked to participate. Informed consent was obtained from 95 women, of whom 46 were randomized to treatment with metronidazole tablets, 400 mg 1 hour before abortion, 400 mg 5 hours after abortion, and 400 mg 8 hours after. Forty-nine women were randomized to similar placebo treatment. Twenty-two women were excluded from the trial because they failed to follow the protocol. Of the remaining 73, 38 belonged to the treatment group and 35 to the placebo group.

The abortions were all performed under general anaesthesia by dilatation with Hegars dilators and vacuum aspiration, the women were discharged the same day. Two weeks later they came for follow-up, including a pelvic examination, in the out-patient departments. All women were instructed to contact the departments if complications occurred. If the women were seen in the departments before follow-up visit a diagnosis of pelvic infection required at least two of the following four findings: (1) a temperature of at least 38.0 °C measured in the department, (2) at least a moderate tenderness of the uterus and/or the parametrium, (3) tender adnexal masses and (4) pathologic vaginal discharge or bleeding.

At the 2 week follow-up visit a diagnosis of post-abortal infection demanded that at least three of the following four symptoms had been present: (1) a temperature of at least 38.0 °C for 24 hours, (2) continued pelvic pain, (3) pathologic vaginal discharge or bleeding, and (4) malaise together with at least one of the following two objective findings: (a) moderate uterine tenderness and (b) at least moderate tenderness of the parametrium or tender adnexal masses.

The randomization of the women with regard to variable age, gestational age, number of spontaneous and induced abortions and births showed no significant differences, and the distribution of antibiotics/placebo among the excluded 22 women did not deviate from the distribution among the 73 participating women.

In the treatment group seven women contracted a post-abortal pelvic infection, and in the placebo group eight women acquired infection. This difference is not significant.

Among the 15 women with infection, three were re-evacuated because of a clinical suspicion of retained tissue. If these three were all excluded, 11% of the women in the treatment group had a post-abortal infection. This is still a non-significant difference compared to the placebo group.

The age of the women, number of spontaneous and induced abortions and number of births did not significantly influence the rate of infection, whereas the gestational age 11-12 weeks did. The effect of treatment was, however, not correlated to this variable.

The present study has confirmed that women with a history of PID and women at gestational age 11-12 weeks carry a risk of contracting post-abortal pelvic infection at a rate justifying prophylactic antibiotics. As the study was designed to include 135 women, the question whether short term metronidazole prophylaxis is effective in reducing the frequency of post-abortal infection cannot be answered with certainty until the conclusion of the trial.

31
Coagulation methods for tubal sterilization – proved in animal model

H.-H. RIEDEL AND K. SEMM

INTRODUCTION

Morphologic and endocrine studies on 370 New Zealand white rabbits were performed from 1980 to 1982, in order to systematically evaluate the extent of the coagulated area following the use of the mono- and bipolar high-frequency technique, the endocoagulation procedure and the CO_2 laser coagulation method, and to prove if there are any changes in hormonal levels following the use of these different techniques.

RESULTS

Through the use of unipolar high-frequency coagulation extensive destruction of the uterine horns and the surrounding mesosalpingeal tissue occurred after a coagulation time of only 10 s.

During laparotomy 1–4 weeks after unipolar high-frequency coagulation, the majority of the tissue found was necrotic scar tissue, whereas after 8–12 weeks the uterine horns consisted mainly of thin, cordlike fibrous tissue. Moreover, considerable destruction of the mesosalpingeal tissue was confirmed.

With application to the bipolar coagulation technique, in which we used the coagulation forceps developed by Hirsch, the production of smoke was significantly reduced, and the destruction of tissue much more localized. Examinations following bilateral coagulation after 4–12 weeks showed a destroyed mesosalpingeal area (approximately 1–2 cm in size) and a swelling of the distal uterine horns that was comparable to a hydrosalpinx.

With a special group of 12 rabbits sterilized by the bipolar high-frequency technique at a current of 7.3 or 10 watt for 10 s, it could be demonstrated macroscopically and histologically that after 12 weeks recanalization of the uterine horns had started or already taken place in five cases (41.7%).

Rabbits coagulated by CO_2 laser on the distal uterine horns were examined following relaparotomy 4 or 12 weeks later. Macroscopic and enzyme histo-chemical studies showed that initial or complete recanalization had occurred in 8 out of 23 cases (34.8%).

As was demonstrated following laparotomy, macroscopically with exact measurement of the destroyed region and later clearly shown by histological, histochemical, electron microscopic examinations and special plastination techniques, the extent of tissue destruction during coagulation by endocoagu-lation or bipolar high-frequency techniques operated at lower coagulation currents was insignificant compared to the destruction caused by monopolar high-frequency technique.

In our department, progesterone levels were determined in 149 New Zealand rabbits before and after stimulation with 50 IU HCG i.v. All the rabbits used for the endocrine studies were held during the pre- and post-operative phases in individual cages. Blood samples from a marginal vein in the ear were taken 4 weeks before operation and 8 weeks after coagulation of the distal uterine horns by using the different coagulation techniques. At the end of this period, the rabbits were stimulated by injecting 50 IU HCG i.v. in order to provoke a pseudopregnancy. During this post-stimulation phase blood samples were taken twice a week, on day 4, 7, 11, 14, 16, 20 and 25.

After stimulation of the animals, with 50 IU HCG i.v., the control group showed a clear rise in average progesterone levels of 12.69 ± 6.02 ng/ml up to the 11th day of pseudopregnancy, followed by a gradual decrease in concen-trations, returning to basal levels at days 14–25. The hormonal reaction of rabbits to monopolar high-frequency coagulation of the distal uterine horns were particularly interesting. Although the average basal progesterone concen-trations were nearly identical in all groups, the progesterone concentrations after stimulation were clearly lower in the two groups of animals coagulated by using the monopolar coagulation technique than in the other groups.

At monopolar coagulation currents of 32 and 68 watt the average pro-gesterone concentrations on day 11 of 7.84 ± 1.68 and 7.66 ± 2.8 ng/ml, respect-ively, were significantly lower than control levels. Similar differences were also evident on days 4, 7, 14 and 16 (Figure 1).

DISCUSSION

As we have shown in the rabbit system, by limiting coagulation, i.e. endo- or laser coagulation, the ateria uterina will remain intact; therefore, significant changes in postoperative hormone concentrations are not to be expected.

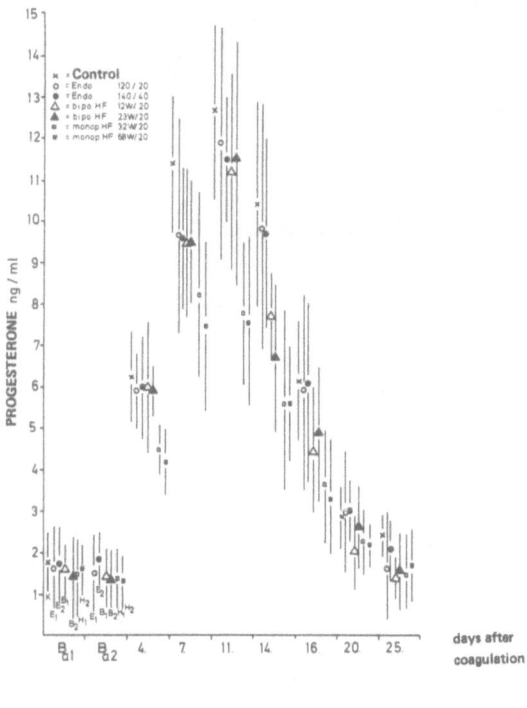

Figure 1 Progesterone levels after coagulation of uterine horns

Differences in the extent of the coagulated zone could not be correlated with the experience of the surgeons, however, it was dependent on the coagulation temperature reached by the tissue and the coagulation time.

As we have demonstrated through numerous enzyme histochemical examinations within the human and rabbit model, at temperatures over 57°C a denaturation of the thermo-labile proteins of enzyme systems occurs, causing a destruction of a tissue area much greater than the primary pale white zone viewed during pelviscopy. During the application of the high-frequency current technique for tubal sterilization, we repeatedly showed that the tissue temperature reached cannot be predicted, since the temperatures are dependent not only on the preset coagulation current of the instrument but on the specific tissue resistance, as well[1].

While the major blood supply between the uterine horns, tubes and ovaries in the rabbit and some other species flow through vessels located deeper in the mesosalpinx than, for example in human fallopian tubes, it is possible in these

181

animals to perform salpingectomies without significantly affecting the blood and nerve supplies.

No definite conclusion regarding the effect of different sterilization techniques on ovarian metabolisms can, therefore, be drawn from these experiments.

Reference

1. Kastendieck, E. and Mestwerdt, W. (1973). Tierexperimentelle und klinische Aspekte zur Technik der laparoskopischen Tubensterilisation. *Geburtsh. Frauenheilkunde*, 33, 971

32
Pregnancy rates after laparoscopic tubal sterilization by means of mechanical and coagulating techniques

H. FRANGENHEIM

Whoever wishes to learn or improve his technique of laparoscopic tubal sterilization will have to decide which method is the most safe and suitable for his own particular situation.

Basically he will have to decide between two major groups of techniques for achieving tubal occlusion, i.e. mechanical or coagulating techniques. It is the purpose of this paper to offer practical advice according to our present medical knowledge.

I want to refrain from repeating the evolution of laparoscopic tubal sterilization during the last 30 years. But the greatest variety of techniques was practised in the late 1970s. It is but human and understandable that every physician who developed new tools or techniques will claim his own invention to be the best.

A great amount of statistics issued by the pioneers of laparoscopic tubal sterilization led in the late 1970s to the generally accepted assumption that all practised methods were about equal and comparable as to the rate of subsequent pregnancies. But there seemed to exist differences between the different techniques as to the avoidable risk to the patient.

Now, what is our present understanding of the problem?

COAGULATION

Unipolar high frequency coagulation

This has been largely abandoned due to a number of specific complications.

Table 1 Change in the use of different methods of laparoscopic tubal sterilization, 1979 and 1980

AAGL 1979		AAGL 1980	
High frequency monopolar	25%	High frequency monopolar	8.4%
High frequency bipolar	50%	High frequency bipolar	74.5%
Clips and rings	25%	Clips	1.6%
		Rings	10.1%
Reference: *American Congress on Gynecological Laparoscopy.* Williamsburg, 1980		Others	5.4%
		Reference: AAGL (1980). *Inquiry of the American Society of Gynecological Laparoscopy*	

Thermocoagulation

The propagation of thermocoagulation was mostly limited to Germany, but it was effected with great effort. However, even the most experienced surgeons had to deal with a rate of 7% or more of subsequent spontaneous recanalizations. Even with tubal division at two sites our own failure rate was within the same range. Thus, in our personal opinion, thermocoagulation is not suitable for tubal sterilization. The technique is not even mentioned in the most recent statistical US report.

Bipolar coagulation

The remaining coagulating method of choice is *bipolar coagulation*.

Owing to its high degree of reliability combined with a low risk to the patient the technique is generally accepted. The failure rate of coagulating techniques is 0.03%.

MECHANICAL METHODS

The problem with mechanical techniques resembles that associated with coagulating procedures.

In the late 1970s a considerable number of rather favourable reports were published for sterilization by means of *clips* or *Fallope rings*.

Larger surveys in the early 1980s issued less positive results.

Clips

From the most recent international publications I have collected the major statistical reports concerning the failure rates of clip sterilization. The published figures range between 5 and 25%.

What is the reason for the high failure rates?

Is it the technique itself?
Is it the size of the clip?
Is it the compression of tubal tissue in between the clip?
Is it necrosis owing to tissue compression?
Is it rejection of a foreign body?

A definite answer will be hard to find.

In this context there is an interesting study done by Mehta in India. It shows the high tendency of the fallopian tube to rid itself of foreign bodies. In about 180 women Mehia performed post partum tubal ligation by means of non-absorbable suture material. Subsequently, a number of these ligatures cut completely through the tubal wall. Within a short time 30% of spontaneous tubal recanalizations could be demonstrated by hysterosalpingography. Why should the same not happen after clip application – rejection of the clip and subsequent spontaneous tubal recanalization? The analogy cannot be denied.

Fallope rings

Looking over the last statistical report of the AAGL, the application of Fallope rings seems to be more widely accepted than tubal ligation by means of clips. In Europe however, Fallope rings have not found such a high number of supporters. The reason is not known. Different from the situation seen with clips, failures of Fallope rings seem to be more inherent to beginner problems with the technique and to originally deficient material. Failure rates in the literature range from 0.3 to 2%.

REFERTILIZATION

In our opinion eventual refertilization should not be the deciding factor for one or other techniques of tubal sterilization. We think tubal sterilization should be offered and performed as a definitive method of contraception. The relatively high number of refertilizations published by microsurgeons such as Frantzen, Hepp and Winston show that most probably the indications for those sterilizations were set after insufficient counselling by the physician and inadequate evaluation of the consequences for the patient. We hope these figures are not representative for the total number of tubal sterilizations.

POST-PARTUM OR INTERVAL STERILIZATION

Sterilizations after delivery or abortion show a higher failure rate than interval sterilizations.

Table 2 Failure rate of different methods of laparoscopic tubal sterilization

I. *Coagulating methods*	
High frequency:	
Monopolar	0.02%
Bipolar	0.02%
Thermo- (heat) coagulation:	
Spontaneous tubal	5.0%
Recanalization	bis 15.0%
II. *Mechanical methods*	
Clips: Hulka	
Secu-Bleier	
Tupla	
Interval sterilization	5.0%
Post partum sterilization	bis 25.0%
Clips: Filshie	
New information*	6000 cases
	no pregnancies
Fallope rings:	
Interval sterilization	0.3%
Post-partum sterilization	1.0%

Personal information *XI. World Congress on Fertility and Sterility*, Dublin

I have received reports of pregnancies even with bipolar tubal sterilization in the immediate post-partum. Thus, interval sterilization is preferable and is the method of choice.

OUT-PATIENT STERILIZATION

If all safety measures are followed and at hand, laparoscopic sterilization can be performed on an outpatient basis.

In this regard the situation will be different from one country to another.

What is the consequence?

In a free market only what is required and what is of good quality will be accepted and survive. This is no different to laparoscopic tubal sterilization. The annual statistical reports of our American colleagues reveal a constant shifting between the different methods of sterilization. Bipolar coagulation is preferred on a large scale. Thermocoagulation (which has been propagated in Germany) is not being practised. Amongst the mechanical methods Fallope rings are gaining and clips are loosing ground.

This natural selection should not be underestimated. For safety sake I cannot but recommend bipolar coagulation for our countries. Tubal division does not lower the failure rate. However, in most cases I personally take a biopsy from the coagulated tube, in order to be able to prove that the tubes have indeed been coagulated, in case of an eventual pregnancy after sterilization.

CONCLUSION

For several years the safety and reliability of different methods of laparoscopic tubal sterilization have remained relatively obscure.

Larger statistics reveal bipolar coagulation as the method of choice amongst coagulating techniques, and Fallope rings as the method of choice amongst mechanical techniques; this has been a world wide development or trend. A number of techniques are of historical interest. They should be remembered as steps on the way to the laparoscopic procedures of today, but abandoned in practice.

Table 1 Laparoscopies 1970–1979

Diagnostic	3640
Sterilizations	2067
Total	5707

Table 2 Pregnancies after laparoscopic tubal sterilization 1970–1979

Personal results $n = 2067$

Technique	n	Pregnancies (%)
HF monopolar	574	2 (0.3%)
HF bipolar	1115	1 (0.08%)
Thermo (endo)	172	7 (4.1%)
Fallope rings	28	2 (7.1%)
Clips	170	6 (3.5%)
Tantalum clips (no longer in use)	27	12 (44.4%)
Mechanical methods total (Tant. clips excluded)	198	8 (4.0%)
HF methods total	1689	3 (0.17%)

33
Acceptability of laparoscopic tubal ligation by Fallope ring when available among other family planning methods in rural Egypt

EL S. ETMAN

Laparoscopic tubal ligation by Fallope ring has been available in a few areas of rural Egypt for the last 5 years. It was essential to evaluate the acceptability of such a method of permanent contraception when easily available among other contraceptives.

A village near Mehalla El Kubra, Egypt, was chosen for this study. This village has a rural health unit and a family planning centre which has been in existence for the last 10 years. Pills and IUDs have been available from the start.

Laparoscopic Fallope ring tubal ligation has been available to the women in this village for the last 5 years. The operation was done free of charge in Misr Company's Hospital at Mehalla El Kubra, 7 km away from that village. After 5 years, 108 women had accepted tubal ligation, forming a percentage of 17.5% among acceptors of FP methods in that village. The other methods used are shown in Table 1.

Table 1

Method	No. accepting	% Family planners
Pills	263	42.83
IUDs	243	39.58
Tubal ligation	108	17.59
Total	614	100.00

The number of women in the fertile age in this village is 1078, and of those 614 women practise family planning by all methods (56.95%). Relation between age of women and choice of method reflected the following picture:

For all methods: the maximum acceptability is amongst the age group between 35-39 years followed by 40-44 years group as shown in Table 2.

Table 2 Acceptability of FP amongst different age groups

Age group	Number of women	% Fertile women	No. of planners	% among planners	% of family planning among each group
15–19	61	5.66	—	—	—
20–24	233	21.61	38	6.18	16.30
25–29	256	23.74	129	21.00	50.39
30–34	177	16.43	139	22.60	78.53
35–39	260	24.12	238	38.70	91.53
40–44	81	7.52	70	11.52	86.41
>45	10	0.92	—	—	—
Total	1078	100	614	100	

Among the group who chose pills: the maximum acceptability was in age group of 25-29 followed by 30-34 years group.

As regards the number of children, acceptability was maximum among those who have three children, followed by those with two children, as indicated in Table 3.

Table 3

| Age group | No. of Children | | | | | | | |
	1	2	3	4	5	6	7	Total
19–24	1	24	8					33
25–29	5	36	46	22	3	—	—	112
30–34	—	8	11	25	12	2	—	58
35–39	—	6	10	9	13	13	2	53
40–44	—	—	—	1	3	1	2	7
>	—	—	—	—	—	—	—	—
Total	6	74	75	57	31	16	4	263

Among IUD users: acceptability was maximum in 35-39 age group followed by 30-34 group. As regards the number of children, it was maximum among those who have four children, followed by those with five children as shown in Table 4.

Table 4

Age group	No. of Children							Total
	1	2	3	4	5	6	7	
15–24	—	1	1	—	—	—	—	2
25–29	—	2	5	5	3	—	—	15
30–34	1	1	16	21	15	3	1	58
35–39	—	4	22	49	34	25	5	139
40–44	2	6	4	5	5	5	2	29
Total	3	14	48	80	57	33	8	243

Among laparoscopic tubal ligation group: the maximum age group preferring this method is 35–39 years, followed by age group 40–44.

Regarding the number of children, the maximum is among those with four children, followed by five children as shown in Table 5.

Table 5

Age group	No. of Children							Total
	1	2	3	4	5	6	7	
19–24	—	—	—	—	—	—	—	—
25–29	—	—	—	2	—	—	—	2
30–34	—	2	3	5	6	—	—	16
35–39	—	3	5	15	15	14	7	59
40–44	—	1	10	9	2	2	5	2
>45	—	—	—	2	—	—	—	2
Total	—	6	18	33	23	16	12	108

CONCLUSION

(1) It is clear that a good percentage accepted laparoscopic tubal ligation when easily available, reaching 17%.

(2) There is a difference in age group and number of children for acceptance of each method. Tubal ligation is preferred by women of higher age and higher parity, especially when compared to pill users.

(3) In another village not given the privilege of laparoscopic Fallope ring sterilization, only 2% of planners have had sterilization, although the two villages are of nearly the same socio–economic group, and the same total percentage of acceptability to FP methods.

191

34
Men's attitude in Israel towards sterilization by vasectomy

S. DEGANI, K. DE VRIES, I. EIBSCHITZ, Z. LEVITAN AND M. SHARF

INTRODUCTION

Male sterilization by vasectomy is gaining acceptance throughout the Western world. The procedure is considered convenient, inexpensive and reliable[1], but is still not popular in Israel.

PATIENTS AND METHODS

One hundred men, whose wives delivered in 100 consecutive deliveries in the Rothschild University Hospital, were questioned about their attitude towards male sterilization by vasectomy. The questionnaire contained questions about methods of contraception and their failures, knowledge about methods of sterilization and desired size of family.

RESULTS

Ages: 63% of those interviewed were in the age group 25–35 years
Ethnic group: 70% were Jews (38% Ashkenazi, 28% Sepharadic, 4% mixed);
             22% were Arabs (16% Muslims, 6% Christians); 8% were
             Druze
Religiosity: 13% religious, 37% traditional and 50% non-religious

Number of children: The desired number of children is 3–4 in all ethnic groups.

Various contraceptive methods were used in 68 couples out of the 100 interviewed. Some couples used more than one method.

193

Table 1   Number of children at home and desired number of children

			No. of children				
	1	2	3	4	5	6	>6
No. of men with actual no. of children	28	26	27	4	5	4	6
No. of men with desired no. of children	0	7	15	26	8	6	8

Table 2

Contraceptive method	No. of users	Failure
Pills	29	5
IUD	23	5
Knaus–Ogino	8	2
Foam	3	0
Diaphragm	2	2
Condom	18	0
Coitus interruptus	25	8

Responsibility for method of family planning:

14% thought that the female should be responsible,

4% thought that the male should be responsible,

82% thought that both, male and female, should be responsible.

Interestingly, of these 82 males, 36 would agree to female (tubal) sterilization, but only 14 to male sterilization.

Knowledge about and attitude towards vasectomy: 53 knew about the possibility of male sterilization. 15 of those interviewed would agree to undergo the procedure after completing their family, and 47 would agree to female sterilization!!

The Causes for rejecting male sterilization:

Fear of irreversibility	– 33%
'Unnatural procedure'	– 15%
Lack of male self-acceptance	– 12%
Fear of the operation	– 12%
Fear of complications	– 5%
Religious objections	– 5%
Not specified	– 3%
Total	85%

No statistical significance was found between the decision about male sterilization and use or failure of any past contraception, age group or number of children, and previous knowledge about the possibility of vasectomy.

DISCUSSION

In the last years, surgical sterilization has gained acceptance throughout the world. Male sterilization has become accepted in developing countries such as India and Korea, and developed countries like the USA.

In 1973, 84% of sterilizations in India were for male sterilization[2]. In 1970, in the USA, among couples having completed their family 9% of the males underwent vasectomy, and 7% of the women tubal ligation[3].

Our study shows that in Israel, the use of male methods of contraception (condom, coitus interruptus) is quite frequent. Many of the husbands (82%) think that responsibility for the contraceptive measures should be mutual, but only 14 of them (18%) would agree to vasectomy, whereas 36 (44%) would agree to tubal sterilization on their wives!!! according to the Roman Catholic and Jewish faith, contraception without a medical indication is forbidden, whereas the Islamic faith allows sterilization with the consent of both partners.

We have the impression that the attitude of the males we interviewed was not so much influenced by religious considerations, but mostly by the fact that societies in the Middle East are patriarchal in nature, and therefore knowledge and consciousness about vasectomy are very limited. We feel that much encouragement and further information are needed to give vasectomy the place it deserves among family planning methods in Israel.

References

1. Silber, S. Z. (1978). *Fertil. Steril.*, **29**, 125
2. Jhaver, P. S. and Ohri, B. B. (1959). *J. Indian Med. Assoc.*, **32**, 193
3. Lee, H. J. (1975). In Sciarra, J. J., Markland, C. and Speidel, J. J. (eds.) *Control of Male fertility*, (New York: Harper Row)

Section 5

Social Aspects

35
Reproductive characteristics of Libyan women

R. SINGH, A. ABUDEJAJA AND M. M. LEGNAIN

INTRODUCTION

Rapid population growth is the most important and urgent matter of our times. The world population increased from 250 million at the beginning of the Christian Era to the current level of 4.5 billion and is estimated at 6 billion by the year 2000 AD. The annual rate of population increase was 0.5% during 19th century, 0.8% during the first half of 20th century, 1.8% in the 1950s, 2.0% in the 1960s, 2.1% between 1970–75 (peak) and declined to 1.9% between 1975–1980[1-3]. All over the world, socio–economic improvements, better nutrition, sanitary reforms and the success over many diseases, epidemics and famines caused a rapid decline in the death rate, and after a variable latent period was followed by a fall in fertility rates with the resultant decline in population growth rates in most regions of the world except in Africa and in the Middle East.

The beginning of the decline in population growth is unprecedented as was the increase which preceded it. The eventual stabilization of population at 10–11 billion or 13–14 billion sometime around the end of next century, depends only on what happens in the field of fertility control during the coming decades. Personal control of reproduction through various contraceptive techniques has achieved very low growth rates in Europe, USA, Canada and Japan. In fact, zero growth rate has been reached in Luxembourg and negative growth rate in German Democratic Republic, Jersey, Monaco and Isle of Man[4] (Table 3). The overall growth rate between 1975–80 was 0.6 for more developed regions, 2.2 for less developed regions, 2.9 for Africa and 3.1 the capita surplus oil exporters in the Arab World including Socialist People's Libyan Arab Jamahiriya (SPLAJ or Libya)[2].

The annual natural increase rate of 3.8% for Libya is one of the highest in the world, next only to 4.5% for Kuwait (Table 4). For the last 2 decades, its economic growth has far exceeded its population growth. The peak of population growth seems to have passed in the year 1975 compared with 1965 for all developing countries and before 1950 for all developed countries, and has not yet been reached for 2 out of 13 of the most populous developing countries (i.e. Bangladesh and Pakistan) and most African countries[2]. The SPLAJs death rate being very low (under 10) since 1964, the decline in growth rate is obviously due to a fall in fertility, and is noteworthy for two reasons. Firstly, it has occurred in the absence of any organized fertility control services and secondly, in the absence of a national policy of population control (rather there are many incentives given by the state for population increase like child allowance and marriage allowance, etc.). On the other hand it has coincided with improvement in conditions, standards of living, education, nutrition, life expectancy and more equitable distribution of the nation's wealth. The present article attempts to describe various corrolates of population growth in the country with special reference to the reproductive characteristics of Libyan women.

MATERIAL AND METHODS

The main sources of data include: (1) the publications of the Secretariat of the Census and Statistical Department, Tripoli, SPLAJ[5-7], (2) Annual Demographic Year Books (1954–1980) of the United Nations[4,8,9], (3) World Health Statistics Annual[10] (1979) and Sixth Report on the World Health Situation[3] of World Health Organization; (4) Staff Working Paper No. 404 (Population and Poverty in the Developing World)[2] and World Development Report[11] (1980) of the World Bank, (5) Statistical Indicators of the Arab World[12] (1970–1979) by the League of Arab States/E.C. for West Asia and; (6) IPPF 1974[13].

The analysis is based, on available information centres, on the fertility levels and trends during the last three decades in the Socialist People's Libyan Arab Jamahiriya, along with changes in the associated and interrelated variables. Comparisons of selected rates are made with other World Regions, Arab World, Capital-surplus oil exporting Arab countries and with countries now reporting extreme values.

RESULTS

Country and its population

Geography

The Socialist People's Libyan Arab Jamahiriya (SPLAJ or Libya) is geographically located on the north coast of Africa along the Mediterranean seashore, and is surrounded by Tunisia and Algeria on the west, the Republics of Chad and

Niger on the south and Egypt and Sudan on the east and southeast. The area of the country is 1759.5 thousand square kilometeres, forming 1.29% of the total land of the globe, and making it the 15th largest country in the world[3]. A large part of the area is comprised of vast expanses of steppes and desert. The part suitable for human habitation is small, and 90% of the population occupies approximately one tenth of the land[5].

Total population

The population of Libya was 1.041 million in 1954, 1.515 million in 1964, 2.282 million in 1973 and is estimated to be 3.300 (Table 1) million in 1983. It has increased by 217% since 1954. The majority (96%) of its population by 1973 was settled[3]. It is a young population comprising 51.4% children under 15 years, 44.3% adults between 15–64 years and 4.2% elderly aged 65 years or more. Thus the age structure of the Libyan population is consistent with developing countries. The proportion of the young population under 15 years of age has rapidly increased from 37.99% in 1954 to 43.6% in 1964 to reach more than half by 1973[4, 8, 9]

Table 1 Population Growth of Libyan Arab Jamahiriya (1954–83)

Year	Population Number (000s)	% Increase since 1954	Birth rate	Death rate	Growth rate (%)	GNP Per Capita (US $)
1954 (census)	1041	—	48.0	22.5	2.55	290
1964 (census)	1515	45.52	23.8	3.9	1.99	640
1973 (census)	2282	119.2	46.9	8.7	3.42	1830
1974	2381	128.7	49.2	8.1	4.11	5960
1978	2824	171.3	43.6	5.6	3.80	6310
1983	3300	217.0	—	—	—	—

Source: Census and Statistical Secretariat, 1980[6]
Population of 1974, 1978 and 1983 are estimates

Female Population: the number of females was 501 235 in 1954, 726 844 in 1964, 994 445 in 1973 and was estimated to be 1 489 144 in 1981[5–7].

The proportion of females increased from 48.1% in 1954 to 48.4 in 1973[4]. The number of Libyan women (15 years or more) was 322 308 in 1954[5], 477 877 in 1973[6] and was estimated to be 716 278 in 1981. Of the total females these formed 61.4% in 1954, 37.9% in 1973[4, 8] and 40.5% in 1981. At present the number of Libyan women of reproductive age group (15–49 years) is estimated to be 603 103 and comprises 40.49% of total females and 84.19% of women aged 15 years or more. Annually, the pool of the reproductive age group's women is increasing by 3.65% due to new entrants to the group of 15–19 years. The number of married women (15 years or more) was 213 807 in 1954, 285 778 in 1964 and 343 902 in 1973, respectively, forming 60.7%, 72.2% and 71.9% of all marriageable females.

Reproductive characteristics

Birth rate

The crude birth rate in Libya was 43% between 1945–49, 38.5% between 1950–54 and 25.1% between 1960–64[4]. It increased to reach the highest level of 48.1% in 1975, and has shown a downward trend since then (Table 1 and Figure 1). The death rate, the second determinant of population growth, was recorded at 22.5% in 1953, 18.3% in 1963 and less than 10 thereafter[4]. Figure 1 shows the effect of fertility on the population growth rate between 1953–78. The number of births has increased by three times during a 15 year period, from 38 798 in 1963 to 11 696 in 1978[4]. Death rate being quite low since 1964, the growth in Libya was solely contributed to by the high birth rate. The high crude birth rate in Libya is consistent with high fertility, and is resulting in rapid population growth in the presence of low crude death rate since 1965.

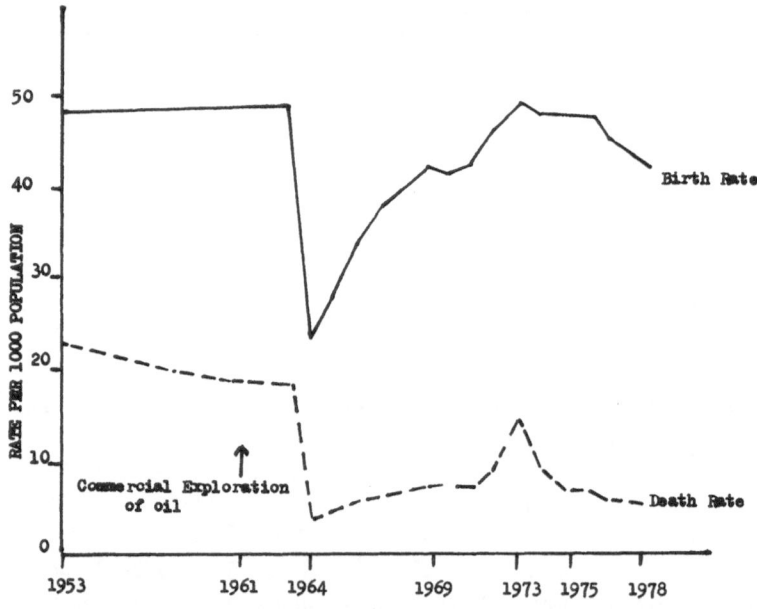

Figure 1 Birth and death rate of Libyan Arab Jamahiriya between 1953–1978

The Libyan population was fortunate when it made the first commercial exploration of mineral oil in 1961[14]. Its real wealth first reached the people in the next few years, and showed its *dramatic impact on the birth* rate when in 1964 it dropped by 26.2 points of its rate in 1963 never to regain that position. 1963–64 was the year when, due to the oil boom, a large number of adults travelled abroad for official, commercial, educational and recreational reasons. People moved from rural areas to towns and cities in search of employment and settlement. Many marriages were postponed for a few years, males were temporarily away from homes and all people were concerned as to how best they could benefit from the oil wealth. It was a year of excitement and population movement.

At present, Libya's population natural increase rate of 3.8% is one of the highest in the world, next only to Kuwait. The only two regions of the world which have recorded a natural increase in the population between 1960/65–1970/80 are Africa and the capital surplus oil exporting Arab countries. The Libyan population passed its pretransition phase before 1950, had in first phase of transition (marked by fits and starts) between 1950–1974, and in 1975 entered the 2nd phase of transition since when its birth rate has started declining. The journey to the third phase with birth and death rates becoming similar at low levels depends upon the fertility behaviour of current and future reproductive couples in the coming years.

General fertility

The general fertility rate (GFR) of Libyan women per 1000 women (15–49 years) has been recorded to be 262.6 in 1953, 231 in 1963, 105.2 in 1964, 224.2 in 1968 and 311.9 in 1973[4]. The oil boom had reduced it by more than half between 1963–64. The latest general fertility of Libyan women is the highest in the world; is 3 times higher than the highest GFR in Europe and is 7.8 times higher than the lowest recorded GFR of 39.7 for German Federal Republic (Table 2). The countries with the highest GFR in other continents are Honduras in North America, Venezuela in South America, Kuwait in Asia and Ireland in Europe (Table 3). The high GFR of Libyan women indicates their high risk of child bearing and their high current fertility levels.

Age specific fertility rate (ASFR)

The age specific fertility of Libyan women is highest in the 20–24 years age group compared to the usual 25–29 years age group in all other countries having the highest GFR in their respective continents, and even in the Federal German Republic – a country with the lowest GFR in the world. A better index of measuring fertility levels is to separate them into different age groups, and in the current study this shows the highest risk of child bearing between

203

Table 2 Selected population and health statistics of Libyan Arab Jamahiriya (1978) compared with world average, and lowest and highest recorded in the world (latest)

	Libyan Arab Jamahiriya	World average	Actual difference from SPLAJ	Lowest in the world	Actual difference from SPLAJ	Highest in the world	Actual difference from SPLAJ
Population density km²	1.9	29.0	27.1	1.0 (Botswana, Namibia, Mauritania, Mongolia)	0.9	4043 (Hong Kong)	4041.1
Birth rate	43.8	31.5	12.3	12.0 (G. F. Rep.)	31.5	52.2 (Niger)	8.4
Death rate	5.6	12.8	7.2	4.3 (Fiji)	1.3	28.1 (Bangladesh)	22.5
Natural increase rate	38.2	17.7	20.5	−5.5 (Isle of Man)	43.7	45 (Kuwait)	3.6
Gross reproduction rate	3.34	2.13	1.21	0.82 (Finland)	2.52	3.55 (Honduras)	0.21
Net reproduction rate	2.52	1.68	0.84	0.80 (Finland)	1.72	3.26 (Kuwait)	0.74
Life expectancy at birth							
Male	51.4	53.9	2.5	35.8 (Bangladesh)	15.6	72.1 (Sweden)	20.7
Female	54.4	56.6	2.2	35.8 (Bangladesh)	18.6	77.1 (Sweden)	22.7
GNP (US $ 1976)	6310	1650	4660	70 (Bhutan)	6310	15480 (Kuwait)	9170
Kilocalories							
Per Capita Per day	2570	2470	100	1710 (Upper Volta)	860	3410 (Iceland)	840
Adult literacy rate	50.1	52	1.5	7 (Ethiopia)	41.4	99 (Western Europe, USA)	50.6
Medical team per							
100 000 population	409.8	349.6	60.2	12.1 (Afghanistan)	397.7	984 (Finland)	574.6

Sources (1) WHO (1980). Sixth Report on the World Health Situation
(2) Demographic Year Book (1980). United Nations, 1980

Table 3 Age specific fertility rates among Libyan Arab Jamahiriya and the countries with highest rates in each continent and Federal German Republic (lowest ASFR in the world)

Age group (years)	AFRICA Libyan Arab Jamahiriya (1973)	NORTH AMERICA Honduras (1974)	ASIA Kuwait (1976)	SOUTH AMERICA Venezuela (1975)	EUROPE Ireland (1977)	Federal German Republic (1977)
All ages	311.9	213.5	207.7	166.0	100.6	39.7
Less than 20	229.4	162.9	107.6	114.9	23.1	17.9
20–24	401.5	306.6	312.4	265.6	139.5	83.2
25–29	350.7	308.3	327.0	250.6	219.4	101.6
30–34	269.3	267.7	236.9	185.5	173.6	53.7
35–39	136.7	195.9	173.3	140.0	106.9	18.6
40–44	59.2	96.9	47.5	60.2	38.5	5.2
>45	25.7	23.4	16.8	12.7	2.6	0.4

Sources (1) United Nations Demographic Year Books (1954–79)
(2) World Survey in Family Planning Needs IPPF 1974

20–24 years. In Libya a married woman is expected to prove her fecundity by child bearing in their first 2 years of contracting a marriage. In fact, a newly married Libyan woman is often happy and satisfied if she has reproduced within the first year of marriage. If not, she is worried in 2nd year, starts consulting doctors in 3rd year, regularly attends local sterility or MCH clinic by 4th year, and travels far and wide to referral centres and hospitals in the hope of child bearing in the 5th and subsequent years. The agony of childlessness is unbearable by the women.

By major regions the highest ASFR is also in the 20–24 years age group in West Africa, Middle East and North Africa compared to 25–29 years in the Indian Ocean area and Western Europe. This in the former regions is due to the cultural expectations, early marriages and, in addition, probably due to low contraception rates in comparison to Indian Ocean areas and Western Europe.

Distribution of births by maternal age and parity

The percentage distribution of births by maternal age in 1978 was 14.6% under 20 years, 43.2% between 20–29 years, 21.9% between 30–39 years and 4.7% at 40 years or more. There were 12.6% women for which maternal age was not recorded. In a recent study at Benghazi in 1980, 53.8% of births occurred to women of 20–29 years of age[15]. In 1973, 8.35% were nulliparous, 23.47% were of low parity (para 1–3), 27.86% of medium parity (para 4–6) and 40.29% were of high parity of 7 or more[4]. In 1980 at Benghazi low parity women were observed to comprise 32.2%, due to the addition of younger women to reproductive population[15]. Nearly one-fifth of births occurred to very young (less than 19 years) or elderly women (40 years or more) and 40% to grand parous women (para 7 or more).

The proportion of child loss in Libya showed a J-shaped curve[15] with maternal age and parity, as also reported both from developed and developing countries[15]. More than 40% of births were of high risk because of high parity of 7 or more.

Total fertility rate (TFR)

The total fertility rate is the average number of children that would be born to women surviving to age 50, if the current ASFR remained constant. TFR of Libyan women has been estimated to be 7.4, which is currently one of the highest in the world (Table 4). It was more than 5 in all Arab countries excluding Tunisia (Table 4), most of Africa and the Indian Ocean[12]. TFR of other capital surplus oil exporting countries is similar to that of Libya, and ranges from 7.2 to 7.3, except for the United Arab Emirates which has a rate of 5.2 (Table 4). The TFR of the whole of Europe and North America is just under 2. The wide varying levels of fertility are due to differences in biological, social and cultural factors operating in different populations.

Table 4 Population vital rates of Libyan Arab Jamahiriya and other capital surplus oil exporting countries

Countries	Crude birth rate (1978)	Crude death rate (1978)	Infant mortality rate (1978)	Natural increase rate (1978)	General fertility rate (latest)	Total fertility rate (latest)	Per capita income (US $) (1976)	Female literacy rate (1970–75)	Couples using contraception (1970)	Life expectancy at birth (1978)
Libyan Arab Jamahiriya	43.6	5.6	42.6	38.0	311.9	7.4	6310	20.1	5	55
Kuwait	51.1	6.1	39.1	45.0	207.17	7.2	15 480	47.0	15	70
Saudi Arabia	51.0	15.0	118.0	36.0	220.8	7.2	4480	5.15	5	53.0
Oman	50.0	17.0	—	31.0	—	7.3	2620	—	5	46.0
Qatar	50.0	20.0	—	30	—	7.2	11 460	—	5	50.0
United Arab Emirates	50.0	18.0	65.0	32.0	—	5.2	14 480	—	—	61.8

Sources (1) League of Arab States/Economic Commission For Western Asia, 1981
(2) Survey of World Needs in Family Planning, IPPF, 1974
(3) Census and Statistical Department, SPLAJ, 1980
(4) WHO, Sixth Report on the World Health Situation, 1980

207

Gross and net reproduction rate

The Gross Reproduction Rate (GRR) is the number of daughters that would be born to women reaching 50 years, if the current fertility rate remained constant. The GFR of Libyan females was 3.34 compared to an average of 2.13, lowest of 0.82 (Finland) and highest of 3.55 (Honduras) in the world (Table 3). The GRR in the Arab World is uniformally high, and ranges from 3 to 3.5[12].

The Net Reproduction Rate (NRR) of Libyan Jamahiriya was 2.52 compared with an average of 1.68, lowest of 0.80 (Finland) and highest of 3.26 (Kuwait) in the world. Thus the population growth rate from one generation to the next is two and half times in Libyan Jamahiriya. The NRR is a better measure of population growth than GRR, as the former takes into account both current fertility as well as mortality rates. The NRR in the Arab countries ranged from 2.2 to 3.3, except in Egypt and Somalia which have an NRR of 1.89[12] (Table 4). Decline in the NRR may occur either due to a decline in ASFRs or an increase in mortality for females.

Fertility attained and lost

The total number of live born children and child losses per woman by current maternal age in 1973 was respectively recorded to be 0.8 and 0.1 under 20 years, 2.4 and 0.3 between 20–24 years, 4.3 and 0.7 between 25–29 years, 5.8 and 1.2 between 30–34 years, 7.0 and 1.7 between 35–39 years, 7.5 and 2.2 between 40–44 years and 7.6 and 2.7 between 45–49 years of age[16]. The childloss per live birth per woman by maternal age nearly tripled from 12.66% under 20 years to 35.23% between 45–49 years.

The average number of children born and lost per every married woman was recorded to be 5.4 and 1.6, respectively, in 1973[16]. High child loss at 40 years or more of maternal age and of para 7 or more has been supported in a recent study at Benghazi[15].

Some correlates of fertility

Standard of living

The standard of living in Libya in terms of levels of literacy in general, life expectancy and upgrading in the average income of all segments of the population has occurred during the last 3 decades. The process of development has in fact accelerated in the last decade, along with a more equitable distribution of wealth and increase in GNP *per capita*. For a large number of developing countries, simple correlation in the 1965–75 fertility decline and *per capita* income in 1970 was only 0.13; but between the decline and adult literacy was 0.70, and between the decline and life expectancy it was 0.76[2]. In Libya, in spite of rapid urban and economic growth, fertility decline was slow, probably due to an increase in the reproductive age group and the unequal distribution of income before 1970.

Infant mortality

Infant mortality in Libya decline dramatically from 300 in 1974 to 61 in 1970[17], and to 42.6 in 1978[18] (Table 4 and Figure 2). Although it is still much higher than for developed countries, it is currently one of the 2nd lowest in the Arab countries as well as in capital surplus oil exporting Arab countries. In Arab countries it usually ranges from 50 to 150 except for 187 in Mauritania[12]. The infant mortality rate in West Africa, North Africa, Middle East and the Indian Ocean in 1970 was more than twice that of Libya, although even now it is still 5 times higher than the lowest reported for Sweden (8), Denmark (7.9), Iceland (7.7)[10]. It is also more than 2.5 times higher than the German Federal Republic which has the lowest fertility rate in the world[10].

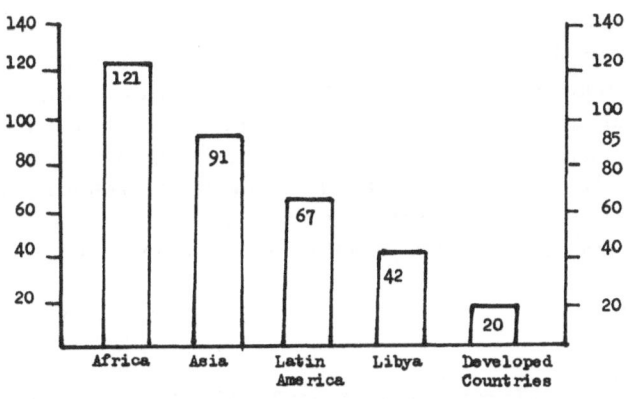

Source: POPULATION REFERENCE BUREAU

Figure 2   Infant mortality rate of Libyan Arab Jamahiriya and world by regions (1982)

Female education

Female literacy bears one of the strongest and most consistently negative relationship to fertility. The female literacy was 12.2% in 1959, 20.1% in 1973 in Libya, and is currently expected to be around more than 60%. The proportion of females among the school population was 44.6% during 1978/79 academic year[5]. The student enrolment since 1975 is almost equal for both sexes. Female literacy ranged from 5 to 50% in most Arab countries, except in the Lebanon which had a female literacy rate of 86% in 1979[12]. General adult literacy in Libya in 1973 was 51.1 being 41.4 points higher than the lowest reported for Ethiopia (7) and 50.6 points less than the highest for Western Europe and USA (Table 2).

Life expectancy

Life expectancy at birth in Libya is now 55 years. It ranges from 50 to 65 in most Arab countries except Yemen, Mauritania, Yemen Democratic Republic, Sudan and Oman which have a life expectancy between 38.3–46 and that of Kuwait of 70, being the highest in the Arab World[3, 12, 13] (Table 4). The life expectancy of Libyans is 15.6 to 18.6 years higher than the lowest reported for Bangladesh (35.8) and lower by 20.7–22.7 years than Sweden (Male 72.1 and Female 77.1) which has the highest life expectancy in the world (Table 2). The life expectancy in Libya has increased from 42.4 years in 1950–55 to 49.0 between 1960–70 to 52.9 years in 1973 and to 55 years at present[4, 8, 9].

Urbanization and industrialization

Before 1950 most people were engaged in agriculture. In 1973, 36.1% of the people were employed in community, social and personal services, 26.5% in agriculture, hunting, forestry and fishing, 17.6% in transport, storage, construction and communication, 11.2% in manufacturing, whole retail trading, restaurants and hotels and 12.6% in others[5]. The Petrol Industry started in 1961 to be followed by many other manufacturing industries in rapid succession[14, 17].

In 1964, 24.6% of the population was considered urban, which increased to 42.5% in 1973[4], and is currently estimated to be more than 50% of total population.

Income

Libya's gross national product in 1976 was 15 140 million US dollars, being next only to Saudi Arabia in the Arab World[3]. Libyan Jamahiriya's *per capita* GNP in US $ was 6310 in 1976; being number 1 in Africa (Table 2), 4th in the Arab World (Table 4) and 11th throughout the world[3]. Libya's GNP was 3.8 times higher than the world average, 90 times higher than the lowest in the world (Bhutan) and 2.45 times lower than the highest in the world (Table 2). Libya's GNP US $ *per capita* was 290 in 1962, 640 between 1965–69, 1960 in 1970, and 6310 in 1976 (Table 1). The present standard of living in modern Libya is due to the unprecedented wealth that the discovery of oil has brought to the nation. In fact Libya has very rapidly recovered from the ravages of the 1939–45 war and its disrupted and underdeveloped state[14]. In Libya and other capital surplus oil exporting Arab countries population growth and economic growth have gone hand-in-hand. Before 1970 there were enormous disparities in the wealth distribution among various segment of Libya's population. These disparities have been rapidly dissolved since 1970 and more so since 1976 onwards. There has been no private trade or industry being run on employee and employer basis in the country for a number of years.

Age at marriage

The marriage of all females is universal practice in Libya. Of all women between the age of 15–19 in 1973 more than 54% were married, and by 30 years of age only 12.6% remained unmarried[4]. The proportion of married women (among all women age 15 years or more) was 42.2% in 1954, 77.3% in 1964 and 71.9% in 1973. Since the mid-1960s the legal age of marriage for girls and boys, respectively, is 16 and 18 years. In actual practice just 20 years ago the median age for marriage was 15 among girls and 20 among boys, this has recently been observed to have increased to 18 for girls and 24 for boys. The mean age of marriage in most Arab countries appears to be between 20–24 years[12, 13]. Currently the age of marriage for girls has been delayed because most of them are attending schools, have an increased opportunity for work outside their homes and devote time to search for a more suitable match.

Contraception

Around 1970, 5% of couples in Libya were reported to use contraceptive methods compared to 1% in West Africa, 11% in Middle East, North Africa and Indian Ocean, and 66% in Western European countries[13]. In the Arab countries the contraception rate was highest in the Lebanon (25%) and Jordan (25%) followed by Yemen (18.3%), Kuwait (15%), Egypt (14%) and Morocco, Iraq and Algeria (10% in each country)[13]. In 1980 the demand for contraception among Libyan women increased to a point that a regular Family Planning clinic had to be founded at Benghazi in February 1982. The demand was so high that within a year more than 3000 women had registered for contraception in a city of 430 000 inhabitants. Such clinics are expected to grow in magnitude and coverage for reasons of health and welfare for mother and children.

Reasons for decline in fertility in Libya

The possible factors or conditions of past high fertility and those influencing the present reduction are enumerated in Table 5. The desire to control conception is arising out of the recognition of the mounting 'costs', in terms of time and energy which children demand for their overall optimum development and upbringing. Presently, women are taking up jobs outside their homes and increasingly find it difficult to carry on the domestic responsibilities of a large number of children. The cultural factors such as the need for sons and children

Table 5 Factors responsible for high fertility (birth rate) in the past, and decreasing fertility at present in SPLAJ

	High fertility of past	Decreasing fertility of present
Cultural	Perpetuation of tribal name Tradition for large family Source of satisfaction and fulfilment	Nationalistic attitude Preference for smaller families
Biological and social	Early age of marriage Universality of marriage, low cost of marriage Polygamy Extend family system Low literacy (general) Low literacy for women Low status of women Most women worked indoors	Late marriage Costly marriage Monogamy Increase general literacy Increased female literacy Improved status of women More employment for women outside homes
Economic	Traditional work; agriculture, pastoral Children as social security Marriage allowance Low cost of child bearing Child allowance Free education Free medical services Inequality in income distribution Low standard of living Less urbanization	Modern occupation and industrialization High cost of child bearing Equality in income distribution Increased standard of living More urbanization
Health	Poor health High infant and child mortality Low life expectancy	Better health Low infant and child mortality Increased life expectancy
Contraception	Absence of family planning services	Presence of family planning services and supplies

to help on the farm and in old age are slowly losing their stronghold. Motivation to 'quality of life' is one of the variables causing the reduction in family size and hence reducing the population growth rate. Motivated couples reduce their family size, despite the absence of organized government efforts, or of religious support as has been observed to occur in some European countries, both Protestant and Catholic[2, 11, 13]. A substantial decline in IMR also seems to be an important factor in stimulating fertility control in Libya. Initially in Libya fertility decline lagged behind the reduction in infant mortality, but now it appears to be gaining momentum. Such motivations to reduce family size appears to have occurred in most countries undergoing social, technical and economic change, especially when infant and child mortality rates have fallen.

Factors tending to reduce family size

Social factors

The socio–economic conditions, e.g. compulsory schooling, increased female literacy, encouragement and opportunities for women to work outside their homes without child-care assistance (due to a break in joint family system) have discouraged many women from having a large number of children. The woman's role in economic life has influenced the family lifestyle, even sometimes breaking the marriage.

Health factors

The knowledge that children born can be expected to live into adult life, the desire to bring up children to be healthy and well-educated, the wish to retain the physical vitality of the mother and an increase in the knowledge, supplies and services for contraception are influencing the reduction of fertility in the country. Decline in the birth rate and increase in fertility control has been found to be closely connected with such changes as the improvement of health care, the decline of infant mortality and the spread of education, especially for girls[2, 11, 13].

Responsible parenthood

A large number of children strains not only the parents' financial resources but also their emotional, and physical energies. The parents' inability to give adequate attention to each child in large families affects the child's learning and development. The concept of responsible parenthood is emerging in this country, in the light of the increasing educational level of the parents and their elder offsprings, and more emphasis is now placed on the quality of children and thereby of the family, community and the nation. Increasingly the spouses are realizing their multiple responsibilities to each other, to the needs of their

213

current and yet to be born children and to their society and state. Traditional considerations such as their productivity value or a means of parental support in old age is not considered that important, or is considered feasible with few but able and qualified children. Responsible parenthood in Libya implies an optimal pattern of family life and of child bearing, the need to postpone marriage and the first pregnancy until the early 20s, to achieve a reasonable interval between pregnancies, to avoid childbearing in later years, and to promote the family size in accordance with the resources and aspirations of the parents. A small family is being realized as being equally happy or even happier than a large family.

Cost of children

The economic costs of feeding, clothing and upbringing has increased. Large numbers of children also put a strain on the parents' physical and psychological resources, as well as on parents' time used for completing other tasks. Some of the time is taken from employment but much of this time is lost from sleep or leisure, or from following their interests. Increasingly, as the society is developing, this time spent on children appears to be more valuable. As more people are migrating to cities, time and money can be spent on other things. Libyan fertile women are passing through the transition in the value they place in children. On one side there is the decline in the economic assistance that children provide, and on the other an increasing realization, by the parents, that children restrict their own activities or ambitions. Such a transition along with socio-economic development is resulting in a decline in the birthrate. Children are being considered less as an asset than as a drain on their own time and earnings. People's raised incomes make the child's contribution less essential, and induces parents to think more of the quality of the child. Urbanization has abolished the simple jobs children could have done under parental supervision. As couples realise the enormous cost connected with children, and have a way of improving their own future, smaller families are becoming a logical and desired consequence.

Equality in income distribution

In general fertility and income are inversely related. The developed countries have the lowest levels of fertility and mortality and the highest incomes. Libya until now had the highest fertility and 5th lowest crude death rate and 11th highest per capita GNP in the world (Table 2). Saudi Arabia has one of the highest fertility, mortality and income rates[3]. Thus, although income and fertility are closely linked, the former is not the sole determinant of the latter. *Per capita* income has accounted for more than 50% variance both in fertility and mortality[2, 13]. There has been a high fertility and high GNP *per capita* in the

214

case of Libya, Iran and Venezuela[2]. These are considered most probably due to inequality in the distribution of income, and inadequacy of health and educational services. The recent decline in the birth rate in Libya, since 1975, apart from other factors such as the availability of health and education services in recent years, includes a more just and equitable distribution of gross national income.

Future of fertility in Libya

The decline in the number of desired children is likely to be counteracted by the increase in the reproductive population (3.6% women annually reach 15 years of age) and increase in life expectancy. The number of women of child bearing age will continue to increase due to population momentum, and this will tend to increase the number of births.

Compulsory education, rapid urbanization and industrialization, emergence of nuclear families, improved status and employment of women, increased social security and opportunities to higher standards of life have created the desire for small numbers of children and the resultant decline in fertility.

The current fertility decline in Libya is considered to have been catalysed by uniform income levels of population. Future declines in fertility would depend on the continued general improvement in living standards (e.g. education, life expectancy and average incomes of the lower half of the population) and provision of contraceptive services to all segments of population. The progressive growth in capital stocks and surpluses and their investment in capital intensive, manufacturing and supply industries, and agriculture along with investment in human development is likely to lead to a decline in fertility in the coming years. Fertility is expected to decline more as every couple comes to realize that the number of children is a matter of choice, has reasons to choose a small family and becomes aware of ways of limiting fertility.

References

1. Agarwala, S. N. (1977). *India's Population Problems*. 2nd Ed., Tata (Bombay: McGraw Hill)
2. Birdsall, N. (1980). *Population and Poverty in the Developing World. Staff Working Paper* No. 404, p. 97. (Washington DC: The World Bank)
3. WHO. (1980). *Sixth Report on the World Health Situation – Part One Global Analysis*. p. 290. (Geneva: WHO)
4. Demographic Year Book, 1979 (Historical Supplement). (1980). *World Summary*. pp. 157–83. (United Nations, New York: Department of International Economic and Social Affairs)
5. Socialist People's Libyan Arab Jamahiriya. (1973). *Population Census and Summary Data*. p. 32 (Tripoli: Census and Statistical Department)
6. Socialist People's Libyan Arab Jamahiriya. (1980). *17th Vol. of Statistical Abstract of Libya*. p. 256 (Tripoli: Census and Statistical Department)

7. Socialist People's Libyan Arab Jamahiriya. (1980). *Vital Statistics of Socialist People's Libyan Arab Jamahiriya.* p. 70. (Tripoli: Census and Statistical Department)
8. Demographic Year Book. (1965). *World Summary.* pp. 122–7 (United Nations, New York: Department of International Economic and Social Affairs)
9. Demographic Year Book. (1977). World Summary. pp. 151–7 (United Nations, New York: Department of International Economic and Social Affairs)
10. W.H.O. (1979). *World Health Statistical Annual: Vital Statistics and Causes of Death.* p. 520. (Geneva: W.H.O.)
11. World Bank Development Report. (1980). *Poverty and Human Development.* pp. 30–70. (Washington DC: The World Bank)
12. League of Arab States and Economic Commission for Western Asia. (1981). Statistical Indicators of the Arab World for the Period 1970–1979. *E/ECWA/LAS/STAT/Ser G/2* pp. 199
13. International Planned Parenthood Federation. (1974). *Survey of World Needs in Family Planning.* p. 84. (London: IPPF)
14. Blunsum, T. (1968). *LIBYA: The Country and Its People.* (London: Queen Anne Press)
15. Abudejaja, A., Singh, R. and Legnain, M. M. (1983). Reproductive Experience of Libyan Women at Benghazi. *Garyounis Med. J.*, 6, 173–9
16. Ewbank, D. and Wary, J. D. (1980). Public Health and Preventive Medicine. In Last, J. M., Startwell, P. E., Chin, J. and Selikoff, I. J. (eds.) *Population and Public Health.* pp. 1504–48
17. Socialist People's Libyan Arab Jamahiriya. (1979). Health in 10 Years (1969–1979). (Tripoli, SPLAJ: Secretariat of Health)
18. Abudejaja, A., Singh, R. and Khan, M. A. (1981). Trends and Factors of Infant Mortality in Benghazi and Libyan Jamahiriya. *Garyounis Med. J.*, 5, 37

36
Fertility regulation clinic in Libyan Arab Jamahiriya at Benghazi

M. M. LEGNAIN, R. SINGH AND A. PARUCH

INTRODUCTION

In the last few decades contraceptive practice has been growing all over the world, including most developing countries. It ranges from 2.9% practice by at-risk women in West Africa to 80% in North America[1]. Between 1971 and 1976 the rate of contraception in the Middle East and North Africa has been documented as increasing from 10.7% to 18.3%[1]. The most commonly used contraceptive methods in the Middle East and North Africa (82.4% of all methods) are two of the most effective and easy to use or reverse, i.e. the oral pills and intrauterine device (IUD). A trend towards greater contraceptive use has been realized in Libyan Arab Jamahiriya (LAJ) for a number of years. Although the contraceptive rate by reproductive Libyan women (15–49 years) has been estimated to be 5% by IPPF survey, it is now considered an underestimate by many physicians and obstetricians in the country.

In general the contraceptive use throughout the world is greater by those women who are urban residents, educated, gainfully employed and living close to the family planning services and supplies. The women exposed to unwanted pregnancies in LAJ but may become so because they are fecund, sexually active, not using contraceptives or in not having a regular source of such services or supplies. Often when asked in maternity wards, MCH centres or community based clinics, a major proportion of women do not currently want babies, but quite a lesser proportion of these are in fact using an effective contraceptive method. There are some others who have already reached a high parity or have had the desired number of children who need a method to limit or stop

217

childbearing. The availability of contraceptive services and supplies at Benghazi was considered by these authors to be an important factor in facilitating their greater use and protecting more women from the hazard of unsupervized practice.

The authors were concerned that in the absence of a regular convenient, recognized and nearby service of family planning information and supplies, the contraceptive practice was bound to be poor, irregular, hazardous and of unknown efficacy. Therefore, the Fertility Regulation Clinic (FRC) was founded at Al-Keesh Polyclinic – one of the five polyclinics at Benghazi in the Libyan Arab Jamahiriya, on October 4, 1981. The present article presents the biological, reproductive, medical and contraceptive characteristics of representative Libyan women who have availed themselves of the family planning services at Benghazi.

MATERIAL AND METHODS

Study area

At present, Benghazi is the second largest city of the Libyan Arab Jamahiriya. The population of Benghazi is currently estimated to be 430 000, and has increased by six to seven times during the last three decades. It is now a well-designed modern city, having a sports area, well-planned modern university (University of Garyounis) with more than 15 000 students on its rolls. There are five teaching hospitals with indoor facilities for 1850 patients, apart from a network of five polyclinics for primary and secondary care, and MCH centres, health centres and dispensaries for primary or first contact care. A large proportion of women attend MCH centres for antenatal, postnatal and child health care, and at present more than 90% of pregnant women in Benghazi deliver at Al-Jamahiriya Hospital, Benghazi (the only maternity hospital for the city). All health services are run free by the state and MCH centres provide free milk substitutes to infant and haematinics to infants, children and pregnant women.

The fertility regulation clinic

The fertility Regulation Clinic (FRC) was inaugurated on 4th October, 1981 at Al-Keesh Polyclinic, in response to the fact that many women at Benghazi (and still in other parts of LAJ) were on oral contraceptive pills either self-prescribed or prescribed by various doctors, nurses, chemists or neighbours. Thus, specialists in gynaecology and obstetrics were faced with the unscrupulous practice of systemic contraception without any satisfactory monitoring by medical staff.

FRC is geographically located at the Al-Keesh Polyclinic which is one of the five polyclinics in the city currently inhabited by 430 000 people. It provides contraceptive services to married women, and has registered 4880 women in a 2 year period between 4th October 1981 to 14th October 1983. The objectives of the FRC are three-fold in terms of service, education and research in the scientific and social aspects of fertility regulation. The clinic is basically designed to meet existing needs and demands of the reproductive women, to provide family planning information without persuasion, and to protect the health of mother and child by making available free consultation and supplies along with general gynaecological screening and care services. The main features of FRC are:

(1) It has been initiated by the medical professionals to match the actual needs and demands by reproductive women.
(2) It provides family planning information without persuasion or mobilization.
(3) It protects the health of mothers and children.
(4) It provides free contraceptive services and supplies for self motivated couples/women to plan their conceptions well.
(5) It also provides screening services for hypertension, diabetes mellitus, cervical cancer and gynaecological infections to reproductive women.
(6) It has flexibility in providing staff and facilities in accordance with the demands for the contraceptive services.
(7) It confines fertility control services to married women as extra-marital conception is a rare occurrence in the country.
(8) It is hoped to contribute to human welfare, personal freedom in reproduction and quality of life.

The clinic has office space for two specialists, two examination rooms, place for records and storing oral pills, intrauterine devices and has equipment for the sterilization of instruments. The ground floor of the polyclinic has investigation facilities for blood grouping, routine blood tests, urine tests, stool tests and radiography. Specialized investigations such as the examination of cervical smears, culture and sensitivity tests, blood sugar, blood cholesterol, and blood urea, etc. are carried out at the Central Laboratory of the Al-Jamahiriya Hospital, Benghazi. Pregnancy tests if required is done at the Red-Crescent Centre, Benghazi. Cervical smears are carried daily to Al-Jamahiriya Hospital by one of the two nursing staff of the FPC for prompt reporting. The Al-Keesh Polyclinic provides primary and secondary care to the population of about 80 000, and specialist care in psychiatry and neurology to the whole city, and houses one of the MCH centres for the surrounding community.

FRC is located at a strategic place close to the sports area with ample open space facing the Mediterranean sea-coast in the north, and surrounded by well-built housing units. It is well connected by good roads both from the city and outside. The barriers of distance and time are overcome due to the high percentage of motor vehicles owned by most families, relatives and neighbours or by the transport system provided by the state.

The clinic can be reached within 20–30 minutes by motor car from all parts of the municipality. Although it is open to women from the whole of the eastern region of LAJ most women (more than 95%) come from Benghazi. The majority of women are Libyan except for less than 1% of women of other nationalities.

Data collection and analysis

The present study covers 4880 women registered at FRC during first 24 months of its inception (between 4th October 1981 to 14th October 1983). The largest analysis is based on a random sample of 200 women attending FRC from the total number of women registered at the clinic. The results have been compared wherever possible with: (1) randomly selected 100 women as the control group, out of 754 women registered at MCH clinic of Al-Keesh Polyclinic for routine antenatal care during 1982, (2) women who delivered at Al-Jamahiriya Hospital, Benghazi during 1980 and, (3) with Libyan women as recorded in 1973 census.

The present study describes the biological, reproductive, medical and previous contraceptive characteristics and future trends of the women registered at FRC at Benghazi since its inception between 4th October 1981 to 14th October 1983, and likely need of contraception services in future.

RESULTS AND DISCUSSION

Number of women

In the 2 year period since the inception of FRC in 1981, 4880 women have registered, out of an estimated 600 000 reproductive women (15–49 years), living in Benghazi. The number of newly registered women has varied from 166 to 280 from month to month without any discernible trend. The women are advised to attend FRC between day 3–5 of menstrual bleeding so that the doctor could be sure of non-pregnant status. The oral pills are started on the 5th day of menstrual bleeding and an IUD is inserted within 10 days of beginning the last menses. Additionally, women are protected by pills for two cycles to cover the period of any spontaneous expulsion of IUD. In doubt women are given a pregnancy test and supplied with spermicidal cream till a clear diagnosis of pregnancy status is established.

The majority of the women take the contraceptive pill, except 161 women who have an IUD fitted. The rate of IUD acceptance has been increasing for every additional 1000 women registered, from 7 for the first thousand to 12 for the 2nd, 35 for the third and 58 for the 4th thousand.

FERTILITY REGULATION CLINIC AT BENGHAZI

UNIVERSITY OF GARYOUNIS
FACULTY OF MEDICINE
DEPARTMENT OF OBSTETRICS AND GYNAECOLOGY

Clinic Number:
Address:

Name:
Husband's Name & Occupation:

Age:
Date of First Visit:

Reproductive History

D/M/Y : Duration : Alive :Planned : Birth : Pregnancy : Delivery : Puerperium	weight	Toxaemia or Hyperten-sion	Normal or Abnormal	and complications
: of : now : : : : :				
: pregnancy : : : : : :				

:D/M/Y : Duration : Alive : :Planned : Birth : Pregnancy : Delivery : Puerperium
: of : now : : weight : Toxaemia : Normal or : and
: pregnancy : : : : or : Abnormal : complications
: : : : : Hyperten- : :
: : : : : sion : :

GENERAL HISTORY

Lactating now
Headaches
Migrain
Varicose veins
Thrombophlebitis
Jaundice
Allergy
Epilepsy
Contact lenses
Other current illnesses and/or treatment
Other past illnesses and/or operations

FAMILY HISTORY
Diabetes mellitus
Cardio Vascular disease
(including age onset)

MEDICAL NOTES
Previous birth control
Method choosen by patient
If OC or IUD

GYNAECOLOGICAL HISTORY

L M P
Cycle   Previous
               Prestn
Loss   Previous
               Present
Dysmenorrhoea   Yes/No
Premenstrual tension   Yes/No
Fluid retention   Yes/No
Premenstrual depression Yes/No
Discharge
Pelvic infection
Sexual Difficulty
PERSONAL HISTORY
Cigarettes No   day
BLOOD GROUP (if known)
FATHER
MOTHER

Have the risks been explained?   Yes/No
Has the GP been notified?   Yes/No

INITAL EXAMINATION

Introitus
Pelvic floor   - muscle tone
Vaginal walls
Uterus Size   -Small/normal/Bulky
       Position   - AV / RV / Mid
       Mobility
Cervix Healthy
       Erosion
       Cervicitis
Erosion Symp   Yes/No
(if present)
Adnexa
Discharge
Breast
Cervical Smear
Varicose veins
Weight
Urine   BP

DATE	FOLLOW - UP	REMARKS	: LMP	: BP	: Weight	: Breast examination	: Repeat smear	: Initials

221

Age of women

By age distribution, 12% were under 20 years, 27% between 20–24 years, 31% between 25–29 years, 16% between 30–34 years, 13% between 35–39 years and 1% were 40 years old or more. Thus, 70% of the women were younger than 30 years and 30% were aged 30 years or more. The proportion of women under 30 years attending the Maternal and Child Health Clinic at the same Polyclinic was 72%, and those who delivered at Al-Jamahiriya Hospital (during 1980) was 66.6%, which were similar to those attending FRC.

The youngest woman attending FRC was aged 16 years and the oldest was aged 44 years with an average age of 26.23 years. The mean age of women attending ANC was 26.06 years, which was not different from those seeking contraception at FRC.

Therefore, most women attending FRC or MCH centre or Al-Jamahiriya Hospital were young, under 30 years. It was mainly due to there being a younger age pyramid in the Libyan population itself.

Parity

By parity at FRC, 11% women were nulliparous, 40% were of para 1–3, 34% were of para 4–6 and 24% were of para 7 or more. The maximum parity of contraceptive adopters was recorded to be 13 with a mean parity of 4.6. Among the women attending ANC, 28% were nulliparous, 36% were para 1–3, 24% were of para 4–6 and 12% of para 7 or more. The mean parity achieved by women registered at FRC was 4.6, compared with 2.9 by those attending ANC. Thus, women adopting contraception had attained a substantially higher parity before adopting control measures. The average parity reached by those women who delivered at Al-Jamahiriya Hospital during 1980 was 5.0, the average parity per every married woman for the country was 5.4[2]. Thus, although by age the women adopting contraception or undertaking pregnancy were similar, they were found to be quite different by parity.

The women registered at FRC were higher by 1.7 para than those attending ANC, but was much closer to those delivering at Al-Jamahiriya Hospital. Thus, FRC women and those admitted at Al-Jamahiriya Hospital had higher parity levels and some had probably achieved the desired parity. A further study is required to dissect out spacers from stoppers, and to undertake the necessary steps to fulfil their respective needs. Several studies have found that multiparity, especially grand multiparity, carries an increased risk to mothers in terms of mortality and obstetric complications, such as placenta previa, abruptio placentae, malpresentation of fetus, postpartum haemorrhage, anaemia, toxaemia of pregnancy and rupture of uterus[4]. The availability of contraceptive services currently at Benghazi, and in future throughout the country, hopefully will reduce the risk to the mother by reducing the grand multiparity.

Period since last delivery

The interval period since the last delivery was less than 1 month for 15%, less than 12 months for 68%, between 12–23 months for 16%, and 24 months or more for another 16% of women registered at FRC. The time from the last delivery among parous women attending ANC was less than 12 months for 2.7%, 12–23 months for 22.2% and 24 months or more for 75.1%. The average interval among parous women attending FRC and ANC, respectively, was 10.4 and 28.7 months. The contraception adopters although having a higher parity were now much more conscious of controlling their fertility after the last delivery and attended FRC earlier than they could have naturally conceived in the absence of contraception. To be still more effective nearly one-third of the women need to attend at FRC than their present schedule of 12 months or more.

The FRC intends to extend the interval between childbirths as desired by the women. Many studies from developed countries, and some from the less developed countries, have shown an association between short birth intervals and higher relative risk to child health[5]. It is hoped that increased contraception would prolong the birth intervals among Libyan women with the resultant benefit to the health of children and mothers in the absence of the added burden of new pregnancies.

Pregnancy wastage and child loss

The FRC attenders had experienced abortions and stillbirths in 18% of cases, child loss in 11% of cases and abortions as well as child loss in 29% of cases. The average number of abortions and stillbirth per woman was 0.24 and child loss was 0.16. On average a woman who delivered at Al-Jamahiriya Hospital, Benghazi had experienced 0.31 abortions and stillbirths and 0.23 child losses. The child loss per woman by all reproductive age groups in Libya was recorded to be 1.2 in 1973[3]. The pregnancy wastage and child loss has been observed to increase with the increase in parity and maternal age at Benghazi as well as for the whole country. These results are in agreement with observations from other parts of the world[4-6]. The controlled fertility and spaced pregnancies are likely to result in the reduction of pregnancy wastages and child losses among Libyan women in the coming years.

In Libya child loss during infancy per 1000 live births has been documented to reduce from 300 in 1950 to 42 in 1977[7]. The reduction in child loss experience by individual couples and the community, among other factors, appears to have influenced the desire to control fertility and this needs further study at Benghazi and in other parts of Libya.

Health of the woman

Medical history

In the past, 89% of women had one to three caesarean deliveries, and another 4% had a medical or surgical disorder. In 7.1% of cases there was a history of diabetes mellitus (5%), and hypertension in the woman's family.

Gynaecological problems

There were 15% women who had a lactational amenorrhoea, 5% gave a history of dysmenorrhoea and 8% had vaginal discharge. On examination 23% had a moderate to profuse vaginal discharge, 20% had cervicitis or cervical erosion, and in 16% cervical smears showed grade II to III inflammatory changes. The most commonly isolated organism were fungal (candida and monillia) in nature.

Haemoglobin level

The routine laboratory test of percentage blood haemoglobin revealed levels below 10 g in 2% women, 10 g in 12%, 11 g in 23%, 12 g in 31%, 13 g in 15% and 14 g in 17% of women. Therefore on the whole, the women attending FRC were generally not anaemic by WHO standards, having an average haemoglobin of 12.4 g%.

FRC provides an additional opportunity for screening important medical (diabetes and hypertension) and gynaecological health problems (cervical cancer, infections and uterine prolapse), and for establishing various hitherto not available biochemical standards for non-pregnant reproductive Libyan women. The chronic diseases once discovered could be managed by the clinic staff in consultation with other specialists, or referred for management at the existing clinics for specified diseases.

Contraceptive characteristics

Past experience

The registered women at FRC constitute 8% of the total estimated 600 000 reproductive women residing in Benghazi. The national proportion of contraceptive practitioners in LAJ has been estimated to be 5%, as compared to 10% each in Algeria, Morocco and Iraq, 14% in Egypt and 15% each in Kuwait and Iran[6].

Out of 4880 women registered during the first 24 months of the opening of FRC, 38% had previously used a contraceptive method. The contraceptive method used in the past, or at present, has been predominantly the contraceptive pill, as also seen throughout Africa, the Middle East, Western Europe,

Latin America, the Caribbean and South East Asia[6]. The orals and IUDs form 61.5% in East Africa, 87.5% in West Africa, 82.4% in Middle East and North Africa and 38% in the world (excluding USSR and China)[1]. Throughout the Arab World (except Sudan and Iraq) 70 to more than 90% use oral pills or IUDs[1].

Future prospects

The reproductive behaviour of Libyan women, as in other parts of the world, is essentially rational, and children are both joy and asset to them. Couples are currently in the process of changing their natural reproductive behaviour corresponding to the rapidly changing circumstances. They are motivated to space and limit their children as they see the real prospects of health, survival, security and a better life. Awareness of these aspects is surely a factor in the decision to practise contraception since these have been made available, and even earlier when available mostly from chemists. The fertility control services in Jamahiriya when fully developed are likely to achieve the best possible relationship between husband and wife and parents and children to enable them to live in harmony within the broader environment. In LAJ the fertile couples deserve to have the essential knowledge of reproduction, and the source and means of conception regulation which is compatible with their Islamic and ethical principles. Socio–economic factors such as raised incomes, literacy and life expectancy in LAJ has played a major role in the fertility changes, which have been observed in accounting for more than 60% change in most developing countries during the last two decades[8].

Access to family planning services and availability of supplies has also been found to significantly influence the fertility changes in the given populations[8]. Child spacing in LAJ is being designed to avoid unwanted and untimely pregnancies, and its health aspect is acquiring greater importance. Contraception is increasingly needed by those couples where the early emphasis on resumption of cohabitation is losing its force, and bottle feeding is substituting breast feeding practices due to employment or other factors. Child bearing and rearing practices are undergoing changes in this country, with the rapid transformation of a traditional society to the modern one. The need for opening more FRCs is likely to be higher, as an increasing number of women plan their conceptions in accordance with their life styles and complete their desired size of families.

Responsible parenthood in LAJ at present and in the future context implies an optional pattern of family life and of child bearing – the need to postpone marriage and first pregnancy until the early 20s, to achieve a reasonable interval between pregnancies (24–60 months), to avoid bearing in later years (after 35 years) and to promote family size according to the resources and aspirations of parents.

There are apparently no professional, religious or social obstacles to effective contraceptive, and barriers like lack of trained staff, finances and public access to information, services and supplies has been overcome by the present FRC at Benghazi. Further experience and study will be necessary to identify risk groups, effectiveness of contraceptive methods and their adverse reactions, as well as feasibility of starting fertility regulation clinics in other parts of the country.

References

1. International Planned Parenthood Federation. (1978). Special Reports: Unmet Needs. *People*, 5, (3)
2. Abudejaja, A., Singh, R. and Legnain, M. M. (1983). Reproductive Experience of Libyan Women at Benghazi. *Garyounis Med. J.*, 6, (2) (In Press)
3. Socialist People's Libyan Arab Jamahiriya. (1980). *Vital Statistics of Socialist People's Libyan Arab Jamahiriya*, p. 70. (Tripoli: Census and Statistical Department)
4. Omran, A. R. (1976). Review of the Evidence. In *Family Formation Patterns and Health*, pp. 17–49. (Geneva: World Health Organization)
5. Omran, A. R. (1978). Review of the Evidence. An Update. In *Further Studies on Family Formation Patterns and Health*, pp. 17–53. (Geneva: World Health Organization)
6. International Planned Parenthood Federation. (1974). *Survey of World Needs in Family Planning*, p. 84. (London: IPPF)
7. Abudejaja, A., Singh, R. and Khan, M. A. (1981). Trends and Factors of Infant Mortality in Benghazi and Libyan Arab Jamahiriya. *Garyounis Med. J.*, 5, 37
8. World Bank Development Report. (1980). *Poverty and Human Development*, pp. 30–70

37
A family planning survey in Ireland

M. J. O'DOWD AND R. PATTON

SUMMARY

Since the introduction of the Family Planning Act in 1979[1] the number of married couples using Artificial Family Planning (AFP) has doubled. Many experience difficulty, as 24% of family doctors will not prescribe AFP, and only 34% of dispensing chemists stock AFP aids.

Meanwhile Natural Family Planners (NFP), and couples not using any method, have decreased in number.

INTRODUCTION

A Family Planning Act, introduced in 1979, allowed the sale of contraceptives on prescription in Southern Ireland. Prior to that the oral contraceptive was available on prescription only for medical indications.

Other artificial means were not available except in Family Planning Clinics in Dublin and more recently in Galway. The main emphasis throughout the country was on Natural Family Planning.

The purpose of this study was to determine what effect the Act of 1979 had on Family Planning in our predominantly Roman Catholic mid and west of Ireland area. Many patients also complain that family doctors will not prescribe artificial contraceptives, and that dispensing chemists do not stock them. We checked the validity of their complaints.

PATIENTS AND METHODS

Our hospital serves a number of towns and a large rural population. A total of 1000 patients attending post-natal clinics were interviewed from 1980 to 1983, and their intended method of family planning noted. During the survey there were 7980 births of infants over 28 weeks gestation. Among other details the patient's age, parity and social structure was also recorded.

All 73 family doctors serving the area were circulated with a confidential questionnaire and prepaid return envelope. Each was requested to indicate whether they offer family planning advice and of which type; and whether they refer patients for family planning advice.

All 53 dispensing chemists in the area were circulated with confidential enquiry forms, and asked if they stock or dispense artificial or natural family planning aids.

RESULTS

For clarity patient numbers are expressed as percentages of the total interviewed throughout the text.

Age groups: Less than 20 = 1.6%; 21–25 = 13.4%; 26–30 = 49.6%; 31–35 = 21.7%; 36–40 = 12.8%; >40 = 0.9%

Parity groups: 1 = 38%; 2 = 27.6%; 3 = 16.4%; 4 = 8%; 5 = 6.5%; 6 = 1.5%; 7 = 1%; 8 = 0.5%; 9 and 10 = 0.5%.

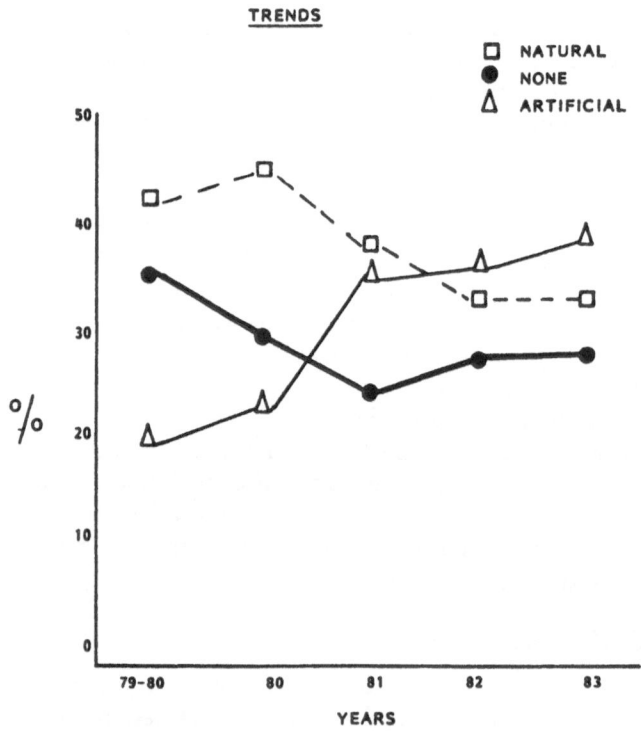

Figure 1 Trends in family planning

Type of family planning used (see Figure 1): This illustrates the trends in natural, artificial and groups not using family planning. AFP almost doubles from 21 to 39%; NFP and the group not using family planning each drop by 10%.

Artificial family planning: In this group the oral contraceptive was the most popular:

| | % popularity | | | | |
	1979	1980	1981	1982	1983
Oral contraceptive	61	86	80	82	76
Condom	3	4	8	8	9
Diaphragm	1	2	2	3	2

There were only a few requests for IUDs, or sterilization.

Natural family planning

| | % popularity | | |
	Billings mucus technique	Rhythm	Temp.
1980	80	14	6
1981	77	14	6
1982	77	12	8
1983	74	20	10

Age by choice of contraception (i) This compares NFP and AFP as a percentage of the total group of 1000 patients.
AFP: 21–25 y = 8%; 26–30 = 22%; 31–35 = 5%; 36–40 = 2%; over 40 = 1%.
NFP: 21–25 y = 9%; 26–30 = 32%; 31–35 = 14%; 36–40 = 8%; over 40 = 6%.

Age by choice (ii) compares NFP and AFP as percentage in each age group. (see Figure 2). There is a striking increase in the use of NFP over 35 years of age. This is matched by a corresponding fall in the use of AFP, the condom being used almost exclusively from 35 years of age in the latter.

Family doctor questionnaire: 75% of doctors returned their forms. 96% advise, at some time, on family planning. 83% advise on NFP and 76% on AFP. 60% sometimes refer for NFP and 54% for AFP.

Dispensing chemists questionnaire: 57% returned forms. 88% stock oral contraceptives; 25% stock condoms, and 9% stock a mixture of diaphragms, spermicides and IUDs.

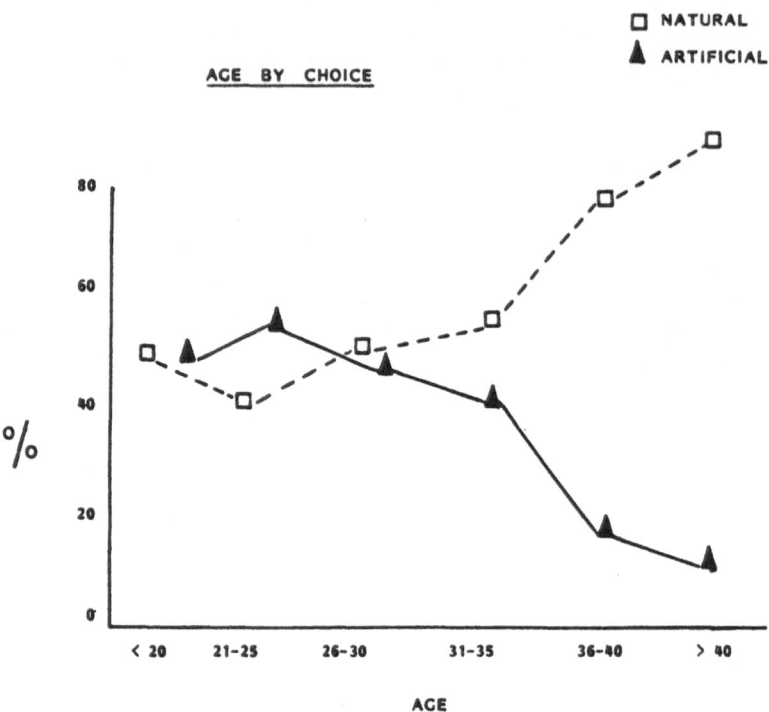

Figure 2 Age by choice of family planning

DISCUSSION

A family planning survey was carried out on 347 patients attending ante-natal clinics in the same hospital who became pregnant prior to introduction of the Act[2]. Our study shows a decrease in NFP from 43% in 1979 to 34% now; and an increase in AFP from 21 to 39%. Patients not using family planning at all decreased from 36 to 28%.

The Mucus (Billings) Technique is used by almost 80% of NF Planners. The oral contraceptive is equally popular in the group of AF Planners. The pill is little used over the age of 35 for AFP, a time when condoms gain in popularity. Conversely, NFP is increasingly popular over the age of 35. The IUD and sterilization were little requested, the latter rarely being available anyway.

Many family doctors will not advise on, or prescribe, AFP, or may want to refer such cases. Most will help with NFP but also will refer to NFP centres.

While 88% of chemists dispense the oral contraceptive, only 25% stock condoms. Many couples with valid prescriptions would, therefore, have to obtain their contraceptives from central FP clinics in Galway and Dublin. This is the trend, with some chemists noting that there is no apparent demand for condoms.

References

1. Health (Family Planning) Act 1979. Government Publications Sale Office. G.P.O. Arcade, Dublin 1.
2. Carr, C. J. (1980). A Family Planning Survey. *Ir. Med. J.*, **73**, 340–41

Section 6

The Male

38
Direct effect of gossypol on the metabolism of rat Leydig cells

G. F. PAZ AND Z. T. HOMONNAI

INTRODUCTION

Gossypol has been shown to be a reversible contraceptive drug that causes azoospermia or severe oligozoospermia. Its mode of action seems to be in damaging spermatogenesis and sperm maturation[1]. Biochemically, gossypol interferes with many enzymatic reactions, including: succinate dehydrogenase, cytochrome oxidase, microsomal oxidase, and uncoupling of oxidative phosphorylation[2]. Gossypol has been shown to have a direct effect on the spermatozoid, exhibiting spermicidal activity[3], possibly due to a direct effect of the drug on the mitochondria and/or pronounced depression of spermatozoal fructose utilization.

Studies on the male endocrine system, following gossypol administration, showed controversial results. In men, testosterone levels and blood chemistry were normal, without any reported loss of libido or potency[4].

In rats, Hadley et al.[5] showed that serum LH and testosterone levels were reduced, and that Leydig cells from treated rats produced less testosterone than controls when incubated with LH. Lin et al.[6] demonstrated clearly in in vivo and in vitro studies that gossypol caused decreased testosterone production by Leydig cells. Thus, a possible direct effect of gossypol on the rat Leydig cells was suggested.

Since gossypol affects enzymes involved in the basal metabolism of cells, Leydig cells are especially sensitive to changes in the energy supply, it is of great interest to study this area. The purpose of the present report is to study the direct effect of gossypol acetic acid on glucose metabolism, oxygen consumption and the viability of isolated interstitial cells from normal male rats.

MATERIALS AND METHODS

Interstitial cells (I-cells) were isolated from the testes of adult male rats (Wister origin) following the method described by Dufau and Catt[7]. Cells were resuspended in TC 199-Hepes and bovine serum albumin (BSA). The viability of the cells was measured by the trypan blue exclusion test (TBE-test). Aliquots of the cell suspension were taken for, 3β-HSD histochemical staining, according to the method of Mendelson et al.[8] Cell counts were performed by the haemocytometer method. Gossypol acetic acid was dissolved in dimethyl-sulphoxide (DMSO) in a stock solution of 50 mg/ml. Gossypol was prepared by dilution with DMSO into concentrations which will be indicated in the results section. 10 μl was added to the cell suspensions, and the tubes incubated for 2 or 3 hours, suspensions were centrifuged and the supernatant taken for the various estimations. Glucose was determined using a Beckman glucometer, oxygen consumption was assessed using the method described elsewhere[9].

Statistical evaluation of the results was performed using the routine methods, and the Student 't' test used for significance of differences.

RESULTS

Gossypol acetic acid decreased glucose utilization when added to final concentrations higher than 100 μg/ml. At 500 μg/ml, gossypol abolished glucose utilization, dramatically. A dose of 10 μg/ml of gossypol had no significant effect on glucose utilization (Table 1). Figure 1 shows the effect of various doses of gossypol on the oxygen consumption of cells, after 30 minutes of incubation, as recorded polarographically and illustrated in the histograms. It is clearly shown that gossypol in doses higher than 10 μg/ml significantly depresses I-cell oxygen consumption.

Table 1 Effect of different doses of gossypol on glucose utilization of isolated interstitial cells from rats incubated for 3 hours. The results are mean ± SEM of 4 runs. Characteristics of interstitial cells at zero time were: concentration, 15×10^6 cells/ml, 3β-HSD stain, 65%, TBE-test 90%

Gossypol (μg/ml)	Glucose utilization (μg glucose/10^6 cells/h)
Control (DMSO)	3.05 ± 0.20
10	2.66 ± 0.24
100	1.83 ± 0.35[a]
250	1.16 ± 0.31[b]
500	0.66 ± 0.52[c]

[a]Significantly decreased, $p < 0.02$; [b]Significantly decreased, $p < 0.001$; [c]Significantly decreased, $p < 0.05$

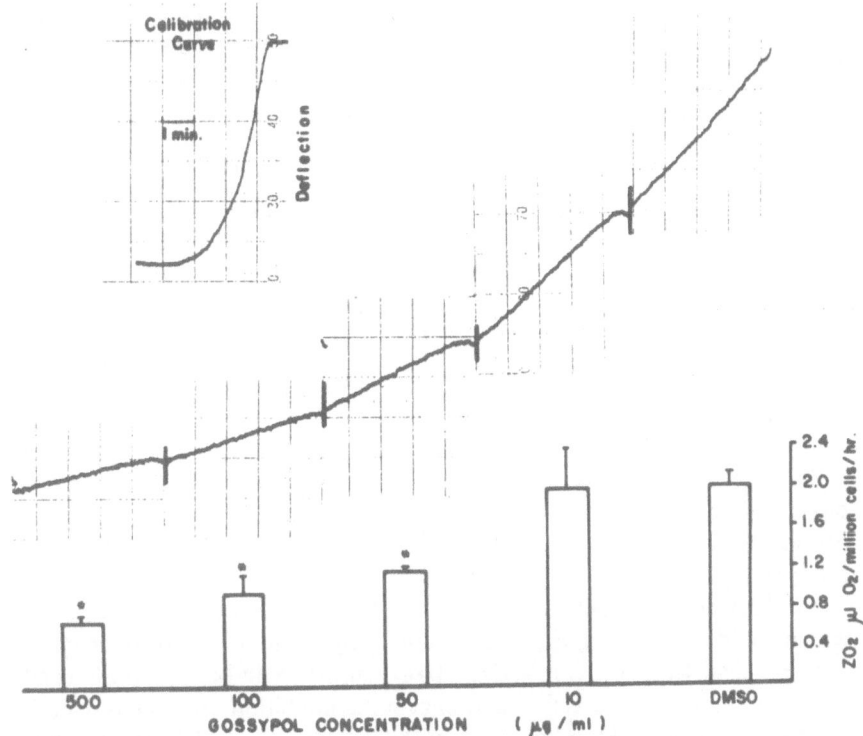

Figure 1 Effect of various doses of gossypol on the oxygen consumption (ZO_2) of isolated interstitial cells, characterized by: concentration, 8.5×10^6 cells/ml; 3β-HSD stain-55%; and TBE-test-90%. Cells were incubated for 30 min and their ZO_2 was recorded for 5 min. The upper part of the figure shows the recording of the polarographic measurements of ZO_2, while the lower part the calculations of the results of 5 runs. The calibration curve was established by the method explained in the text

The effect of gossypol on testosterone secretion of isolated I-cells and cell characteristics are given in Table 2. I-cells responded well to hCG stimulation. Gossypol did not affect testosterone tonic secretion by I-cells, although cell viability and 3β-HSD histochemical stain were depressed.

In order to rule out the possibility that gossypol acetic acid kills the cells by its acidity effects, the pH of the incubation media was measured. Only minor changes were found (Table 2).

DISCUSSION

The present study clearly shows that gossypol acetic acid has a direct effect on isolated interstitial cells of rats. Gossypol significantly depressed the metabolic rate of I-cells; glucose utilization was abolished (initial dose of 100 μg/ml of gossypol). At the same dose, or even less (50 μg/ml), the oxygen consumption was reduced.

237

Table 2 Effect of gossypol on the characteristics of rat isolated interstitial cells (cell concentration 9.5×10^6/ml), and testosterone secretion *in vitro*, under different doses of gossypol. Numbers are mean ± SEM of 5 runs

Treatment	3β-HSD (% stained)	Trypan blue exclusion (% not stained)	pH	Testosterone secretion (ng/10⁶ cells/h)
(0) DMSO (10μl)	50 ± 5	73 ± 0.9	7.51 ± 0.03	0.39 ± 0.029
hCG (25 mIU/ml)	73 ± 4	81 ± 1.5	7.63 ± 0.03	0.60 ± 0.032[a]
gossypol 10 μg/ml	45 ± 4	74 ± 4.5	7.66 ± 0.01	0.46 ± 0.032
gossypol 50 μg/ml	39 ± 5	68 ± 3.7	7.63 ± 0.03	0.46 ± 0.032
gossypol 500 μg/ml	5 ± 3	34 ± 2.8	7.52 ± 0.01	0.34 ± 0.016

[a]Significantly changed, $p < 0.001$

At these doses, the toxicity of gossypol was not pronounced, only in higher doses (500 μg/ml) was the viability of cells decreased. Nevertheless, the 3β-HSD histochemical stain showed a marked diminution when gossypol was added to the isolated cells.

All these activities cannot be attributed to changes in the pH of the media, which could be expected, due to its acetic component. Thus, the toxic effect of gossypol was clearly proven, and can be explained on the basis of its direct effect on the mitochondria of cells[10] and enzymatic inhibition on a large scale[11, 12]. Gossypol is known to have some chelating activity, which can react with cations thus affecting cell activity.

In the rat, some authors showed inhibition of steroidogenesis *in vivo*[5, 6], and *in vitro*[6]. Others failed to show such a change *in vivo*[13], they even showed no change in male accessory sex gland weight or excretions.

In the present study, no effect on steroidogenesis of I-cells could be demonstrated. We suppose that under stimulation of cells, gossypol may cause metabolic changes, which will be reflected in diminished cell activities.

SUMMARY

The direct effect of gossypol acetic acid on collagenase isolated rat interstitial cells was investigated. It was shown that gossypol acetic acid significantly depressed the metabolic rate of the cells. Glucose utilization was abolished by a starting dose of 100 μg/ml. Oxygen consumption of I-cells was reduced even at a smaller dose of gossypol (50 μg/ml). Increasing doses of gossypol caused a marked decrease in the vitality of I-cells, and a dramatic drop in histochemical staining for 3β-HSD. In cultures of I-cells not stimulated by hCG, gossypol did not affect the tonic slow release of testosterone.

Referenes

1. Prasad, M. R. N. and Diczfalusy, E. (1982). Gossypol. *Int. J. Androl. (Suppl.)*, **5**, 53
2. Tso, W. W. and Lee, C. S. (1981). Effect of gossypol on boar spermatozoa *in vitro*. *Arch. Androl.*, **7**, 85
3. Waller, D. P., Fong, H. H. S., Cordell, C. F. and Soejarto, D. D. (1981). Antifertility effects of gossypol and its impurities on male hamsters. *Contraception*, **23**, 653
4. Coutinho, E., Segal, S. J. and Melo, J. F. (1982). Biphasic action of gossypol in men. *Fertil. Steril.*, (In press)
5. Hadley, M. A., Lin, C. Y. and Dym, M. (1981). Effects of gossypol on the reproductive system of the male rats. *J. Androl.*, **2**, 190
6. Lin, J., Murono, E. P., Osterman, J., Nankin, H. R. and Couleson, P. B. (1981). Gossypol inhibits testicular steroidogenesis. *Fertil. Steril.*, **35**, 563
7. Dufau, M. L. and Catt, K. J. (1975). Gonadotropic stimulation of interstitial cell function of rat testis *in vitro*. *Methods Enzymol.*, **39**, 252
8. Mendelson, C., Dufau, M. and Catt, K. (1975). Gonadotropin binding and stimulation of cyclic adenosine 3',5' monophosphate and testosterone production in isolated Leydig cells. *J. Biol. Chem.*, **250**, 8818
9. Frenkel, G., Peterson, R. N. and Freund, M. (1973a). Changes in the metabolism of guinea pig sperm from different segments of the epididymis. *Proc. Soc. Exp. Biol. (NY)*, **143**, 1231
10. Xue, S. P. (1981). Studies on the infertility effects of gossypol, a new contraceptive for males. In Chang, C. F., Griffin, D. and Wollman, A. (eds.) *Symposium on Recent Advances in Fertility Regulation*. September 1980, Beijing (Geneva: Atar)
11. Myers, B. D. and Throneberry, C. O. (1966). Effect of gossypol on some oxidative respiratory enzymes. *Plant Physiol.*, **41**, 787
12. Lee, C. Y. and Malling, H. Y. (1981). Selective inhibition of Sperm – Specific lactate dehydrogenase X by an antifertility agent, gossypol. *Fed. Proc.*, **40**, 718
13. Kalla, N. R., Foo, J. J. W. and Sheth, A. R. (1982). Studies on the male antifertility agent Gossypol acetic acid. V. Effect of Gossypol acetic acid on the fertility of male rats. *Andrologia*, **14**, 492

39
Gossypol as a male oral contraceptive: trial case report

R. MORI, H. HOSHIAI, S. UEHARA, F. NAGAIKE, A. TSUIKI
AND M. SUZUKI

INTRODUCTION

Numerous reports on male contraceptives have been published, but reports as to effectiveness, reversibility and safety are scanty. Many of them describe only success or serious side effects.

Recently, gossypol has been reported to be used in the People's Republic of China as an effective male antifertility agent. Gossypol, a yellowish phenolic compound isolated from the seeds, stem or root of cotton plants, was discovered in the 1950s in China during a mass investigation to determine whether cooking with crude cottonseed oil could lead to infertility in males without causing female infertility. In 1971 an effective antifertility compound, gossypol, was extracted and purified from cottonseed oil.

SUBJECTS AND METHODS

A 35-year-old healthy man, 75 kg body weight and 175 cm in height, volunteered for the study. He had no special past history of illness, and was living with his wife and three children. The volunteer took one tablet containing 20 mg of gossypol daily for 19 days.

Semen analyses, Gn-RH tests, TRH tests and other laboratory examinations were carried out on the day before the start of gossypol administration, and on the 10th and 19th days of the administration period. LH, FSH, PRL and testosterone levels in serum were measured every day during the gossypol administration period and for 10 days after its termination.

RESULTS

Semen analysis

We examined semen volume, percentage of motile spermatozoa, morphological anomalies, sperm density, pH of sperm and the white blood cell count (WBC). (Table 1).

Table 1 Semen analysis

	The day before medication	10th day of medication	19th day of medication	10 days after medication
Semen volume (ml)	7.2	4.6	5.8	6.2
% Spermatozoa motile	60	57	61	62
Morphological anomaly (%)	2	3	2	0
Sperm density (10^6/ml)	76	59	48	86
pH of semen	7.7	7.8	8.1	8.0
WBC	1–2/F	0–1/F	0–1/F	0–1/F

All results except sperm density were constant and within the normal range. The sperm density level gradually decreased from 76×10^6/ml on the day before gossypol administration to 48×10^6/ml on the day after medication. Ten days after the termination of gossypol, the sperm density recovered to its pre-administrative level of 86×10^6/ml. Changes in the levels of four hormones were measured from the day before the initiation of gossypol administration to the 10th day after the termination of medication (Figure 1). After 10 days, LH and

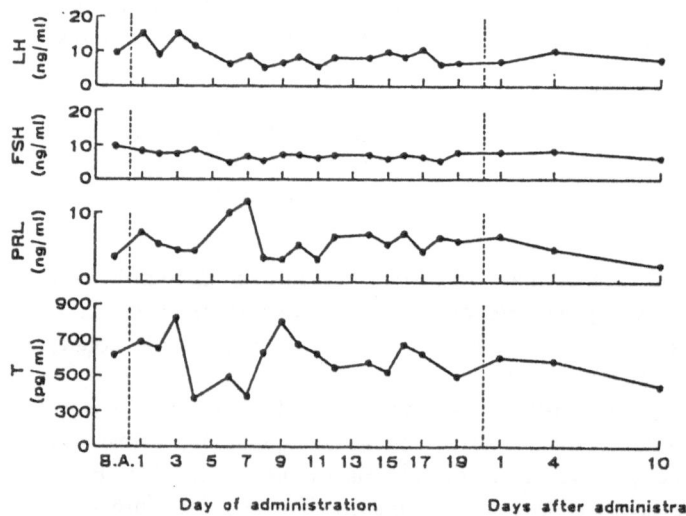

Figure 1 Changes of serum LH, FSH, PRL and testosterone levels during gossypol administration

242

FSH levels were constant at 10.5 ± 5 ng/ml and 8.0 ± 3 ng/ml, respectively. PRL levels varied slightly within normal range. On the 5–7th day of gossypol administration the levels of PRL were a little higher, but after the 8th day of administration, they were almost constant at 2–7 ng/ml. Testosterone levels also varied, and were lower than the premedication level from the 4th to the 8th day of adminstration. On the 9th day, the testosterone level was 795 pg/ml, then gradually decreased to 576 pg/ml on the 10th day of gossypol administration. However, all testosterone levels were within the normal range.

Gn-RH test

Gossypol had no effect on LH and FSH released from the pituitary gland by Gn-RH.

TRH test

The peak of PRL level may be different during gossypol medication, although it is hard to draw a definite conclusion from the result of only one trial case of the TRH test.

CONCLUSIONS

In laboratory findings of the side effects of gossypol medication, the volunteer showed an abnormality in the thymol turbidity test (TTT), creatinine and neutral fat test before gossypol administration. Gossypol medication induced no ill effect according to the laboratory findings. In fact, TTT, creatinine and neutral fat levels improved during gossypol medication. Gossypol showed no acute side effects at the presently used dose of 20 mg/day.

Index